Innovative Technologies and Non-Invasive Procedures in Bariatric Surgery

Jérôme Dargent

Innovative Technologies and Non-Invasive Procedures in Bariatric Surgery

Springer

Jérôme Dargent
Polyclinique Rillieux
Lyon
France

ISBN 978-2-8178-0403-3 ISBN 978-2-8178-0404-0 (eBook)
DOI 10.1007/978-2-8178-0404-0
Springer Paris Heidelberg New York Dordrecht London

Library of Congress Control Number: 2012954870

Printed on acid-free paper

Springer is part of Springer Science+Business Media (www.springer.com)

Principles of a Directory

At first glance, bariatric surgery seems well established in many countries around the world, and gaining popularity along with the continuous increase of the morbidly obese population. Yet the vast majority of the obese population does not take advantage from the surgical possibilities. Clinical research should be oriented towards less invasive procedures that could be accepted by the mainstream. In 2013, most of non-invasive bariatric techniques are not standardized and sufficiently assessed, but they are being constantly upgraded.

The purpose of the 1st and 2nd International Meetings on Non Invasive Bariatric Techniques (Lyon, France, May 13–14, 2011 and April 20–21, 2012; www.noninva-obesity.com) has been to elicit discussion among experts from worldwide, and gather relevant information on new technologies that will make it possible to enlarge the vision of bariatric cares to a growing number of morbid obese and non-morbid obese patients.

The program had been divided into five parts, and established the guidelines for the present directory: (1) Procedures that aim at lowering the "surgical trauma", mostly the single-trocar and the NOTES approaches. They raise important questions. Do we have the instruments we need? Is the upgrade relevant versus the typical lap-approach? (2) Techniques that are available through "natural orifices", the most promising provided they can prove satisfactory and long-standing. (3) New technologies, like neuromodulation. (4) Transversal issues: the role of the anesthesiologist, the cooperation of the gastro-enterologist, etc. (5) Guidelines for the foreseeable evolutions.

Surgical procedures that are well known and accepted in 2012 (gastric bypass, adjustable band, sleeve gastrectomy) were not explicitly addressed as such, but only from the perspective of comparison and confrontation with less invasive procedures.

Figuring out the transition from mini-invasive to non-invasive may be described with the following steps: (1) Picking-up procedures with medium aggressiveness such as SILS and NOTES, as well as parallel concepts like neuro-modulation. (2) Seeking concept similarities: endo-stapling/VBG, endo-sleeve/BPD, endoplication/surgical plication, internal/external bands, etc. (3) Organizing strategies: combining experimental and well-known techniques, stepping up the invasive degree; in this regard, endoscopic redo for failed procedures is a promising direction.

Bariatric surgery is rapidly and highly evolving, and less aggressive procedures are an absolute necessity. Nonetheless, alternatives should be tested in a timely manner, such as stated in the ASMBS recommendations (Statements on emerging endosurgical bariatric interventions, SOARD, 2009).

We chose to pick up interesting and recent abstracts (or the relevant ones) pertaining to each topic; some are quoted in extenso, some are rearranged. An illustration has been provided for most techniques.

ATTENTION: Many if not most of the operations herein described are under scrutiny and/or investigation, with or without the support of major international or national scientific societies. Some of the devices do not have an official approval yet (CE market-approval, FDA acknowledgment), and some have not been tested in humans. Some have even been shut down, but represent an interesting step that can benefit to other techniques. This is a highly evolving field, so please apologize errors and imprecisions. Corrections will be made in the next edition.

Lyon, France Jérôme Dargent

Contents

A

ABILITI® System

(see section "Neuromodulation in Obesity Treatments")

Anaesthesia: Less Invasive Approach in the Obese Patient; Anaesthesiology for Non Invasive Bariatric Surgery

The Opinion of Two Experts

Jan Mulier (Belgium): Brugge-Hospital, Anaesthesiology Department, President of ESPCOP (European Society of peri Operative Care of the Obese Patient)

What are the basis of non Invasive Anaesthesia today? While surgery is moving from less invasive laparoscopy to non invasive natural orifice surgery, anaesthesia is following this move from invasive deep general anaesthesia to less invasive anaesthesia. This means deep neuromuscular block with lighter depth of anaesthesia, lower inflation pressures for laparoscopy but keeping surgical workspace sufficient, opioid free anaesthesia improving the postoperative analgesia, spontaneous breathing with support during pneumoperitoneum, permissive hypercapnia improving oxygen delivery and faster recovery. All these approaches are used today, minimize the peri-operative complications of bariatric anaesthesia and improve the Enhanced Recovery After bariatric Surgery (ERAS).

Although the morbid obese patient is at higher risk, the use of a multimodal technique allows giving a non invasive sedation or a monitored anaesthesia care for a non invasive surgery. As surgeons are moving in this non invasive direction, anaesthesiologists should follow upon their steps to keep their role in the multidisciplinary team.

Ashish C Sinha (USA): Anesthetic Issues in Minimally Invasive Surgery, Ashish C Sinha, Department of Anesthesia, Drexel University College of Medicine,

J. Dargent, *Innovative Technologies and Non-Invasive Procedures in Bariatric Surgery*,
DOI 10.1007/978-2-8178-0404-0_1, © Springer-Verlag France 2013

Hahnemann University Hospital, Philadelphia, USA. President of ISPCOP (International Society for the Perioperative Care of the Obese Patient).

Are there anaesthesia perspective based advantages/disadvantages and challenges when the surgeon prefers a minimal approach? Does it matter (affect outcomes) during the intraoperative or immediate post operative period? Can we speculate to these advantages in the absence of hard data? If there is no hard evidence to these advantages, do we at least have an "expert view point" (or what would an experienced anaesthesia practitioner intuitively feel be advantageous)?

While all minimal approach surgeries have obvious advantages, both to patients and surgeons, in terms of rapid discharge, minimal pain, rapid return to function among others, the degree of advantage to anesthetic care remains to be established. To an anesthesiologist, minimal approach surgery, whether laparoscopic, robotic or NOTES, offer a different set of challenges. It starts from limited access to the patient who may be surrounded by robotic arms with very little approach area left. On the other hand is Trans Oral Robotic Surgery (TORS) where the access to the patients' airway is severely restricted for the anaesthesia provider and the patient's head is the furthest away from the anaesthesia machine and anaesthesist. In this instance, it is difficult to diagnose airway disconnection and then take the necessary rapid corrective action. Another example is the length of surgery, which is especially longer during the first dozen or two cases of that surgeon and also in training centers, where the very nature of practice implies longer surgical times. This comes to a head when at midnight or later the surgeon posts what would be a 20 min open appendectomy as a laparoscopic appendectomy and it takes 60 min of laparoscopic attempts and an additional 20 min when the decision is made to convert it to an open surgery.

The true challenge is to be vigilant to the potential for a vascular mishap as even in the initial trocar placement for laparoscopic surgery when the aperture may create a big enough vascular opening that the initial insufflations of gas causes a venous air embolism (VAE). This of course presents itself in a dramatic fashion with a cardiac arrest! The therapy is a head down position, immediate central access to the right atrium and withdrawal of the air, usually resulting in a good outcome. The other aspect, at least in a case like robotic prostatectomy, is the amount of time spent by the patient in a head-down position. This can result in head and neck swelling, clearly demonstrated by periorbital oedema. In this instance the question is: does the facial swelling reflect airway swelling as well? To extubate or not to extubate, as well as if so, how to do it safely? The leak test can help guide that decision.

On the flip side, to the anaesthesiologist are the advantages of decreased blood loss, at least usually; and a shorter case, at least eventually. Plus, smaller incisions imply less surgical pain and thereby increased patient comfort.

Anti-reflux Endoscopic Procedures

Endoscopic therapy for gastroesophageal reflux disease has been a leading research procedure for 20 years, and has been deemed to possibly replace anti-reflux surgery: e.g. (Oleynikov et al. 2004).

Hopes and expectations have been somewhat unmet, especially toward medications (while surgery itself did not really soar), but this field remains a benchmark to what can be done in bariatric procedures. Various techniques have been described that reinforce the gastro-oesophageal (GE) junction and/or the Lower Esophageal Sphincter (LES). Although most of them have been more or less discarded, many could be (or have been) used for obesity treatment.

The Use of Radio-Frequency

The STRETTA® System (Curon) consists of four radial needles attached to a balloon catheter, and a control module which delivers radiofrequency energy to the tissue. Its goal is to create thermal lesions in the Lower Esophageal Sphincter (LES): as lesions heal, tissue contracts. Technique: Balloon inflation introduces the needles into the esophageal wall; application of microwaves creates thermal energy to heat the tissue. The 6 months Clinical Trial Data have shown a decrease in pH from 10.1 (6.1–14.7) to 6.4 (3.7–12.2), and in LESP (mm Hg) from 15.0 (10.8) to 12.6 (9.4–18.5) (Wolfsen and Richards 2002).

A similar "healing process" has been used in obesity treatment (see section "Safestitch Device").

Non-Circular Injection of Polymers and Circular Injection of a Non Absorbable Polymer

These polymers solidify after injection (e.g. Enteryx®, Boston, Gatekeeper®, idem Medtronic). The Enteryx procedure allowed the injection of a radio-opaque material in order to check for the circularity of the injection. These polymers have been thoroughly evaluated (including carcinogenesis studies), and stem from intra-arterial radiological technology (embolization).

These devices involve strictly the GE junction and have no effect on food intake, except a mild and transient dysphagia in less than 10 % of the cases, which has also been observed in anti-reflux surgery (Mason et al. 2002; Johnson et al. 2003).

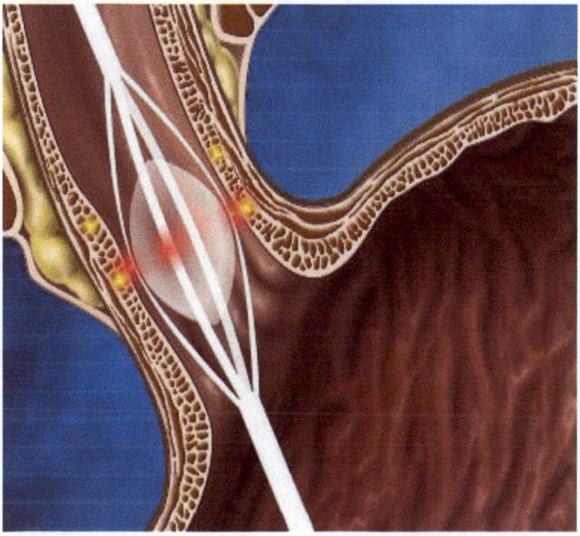

Fig. 1 The Stretta procedure for GERD

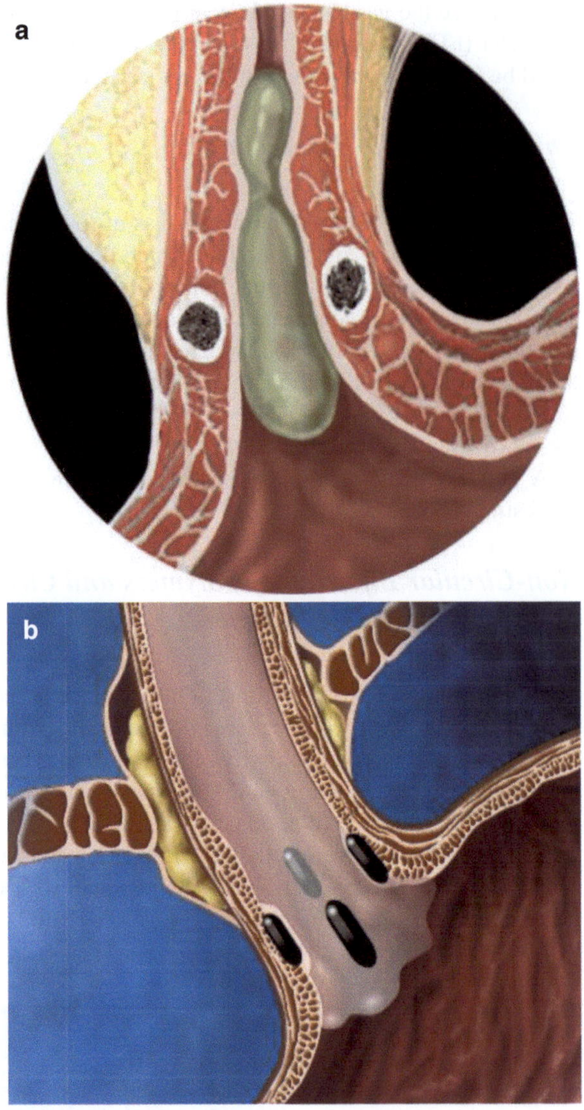

Fig. 2 Circular (**a**) and non circular (**b**) injection at the GE junction for GERD

- **The Gatekeeper® Reflux Repair System**: An expandable hydrogel prosthesis is injected into the submucosa of the LES. Its goal is to act as a bulking agent to enhance the barrier to reflux. Technique: under endoscopic visualization, the dry gel is injected into the wall of the esophagus near the LES and is designed to expand when in contact with moisture.
- **The Enteryx® Procedure**: A biocompatible polymer solution is injected circumferentially into the muscle layer of the LES. Its goal is to improve LES compliance through fibrous encapsulation of the polymer implant. Technique: under endoscopic and fluoroscopic visualization, the polymer is injected into the LES at or below the Z line. At 12-month follow-up, 80.6 % of patients

showed significant improvement in PPI dependency, 71.4 % of patients were off PPIs, and the remaining 9.2 % reduced daily dependence by 50 % or more.

Both these procedures have been abandoned, the concept remaining potentially instrumental.

Absorbable material has also been tested: (O'Connor and Lehman 1988). Such use has also been made in bariatric surgery as an adjuvant (see section "Injection at the GE Junction").

Full-Thickness Gastric Plication

EndoCinch System (Bard®): a suction chamber in the suturing device creates a plication at the level of the LES. Multiple sutures are used to secure the plications. It is designed to create an internal plication of the stomach, and a bulking effect at the GE junction. Technique: it creates two to sixfolds from the lower part of the esophagus to the upper part of the great curvature. Two-year follow-up on 33 patients revealed a 44 % failure rate (defined as the need for PPI therapy or subsequent antireflux surgery): 25 % were completely off medications, 40.6 % were on full dose medications.

The Plicator® System (NDO Surgical) is a reusable plicator instrument and specially designed tissue retractor, with a single-use cartridge containing a suture-based implant. It is designed to create a full-thickness plication, permitting serosa-to-serosa healing and restructuring of the anti-reflux barrier. Technique: the tissue retractor pulls in a full-thickness fold of the gastric wall which is secured with a pre-tied, suture-based implant (Swain and Mills 1986; Martinez-Serna et al 2000; Pleskow et al 2004).

One can see that this kind of procedure is quite similar to the USGI Pose procedure (see section "Transport G-Prox "ROSE" for Re-do After Failed Gastric Bypass

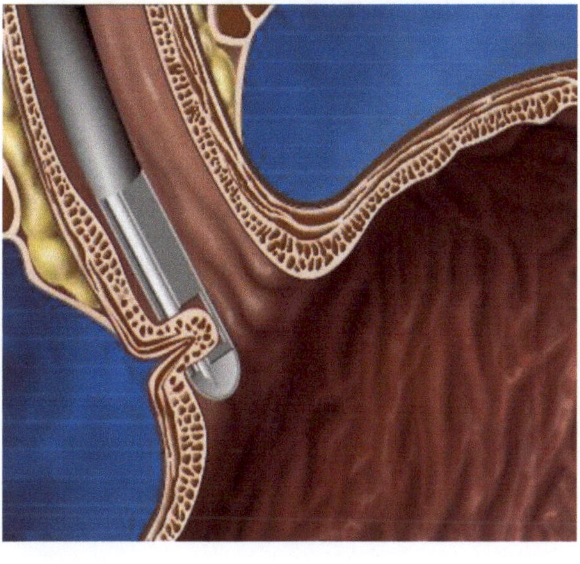

Fig. 3 Endocinch® System for GERD

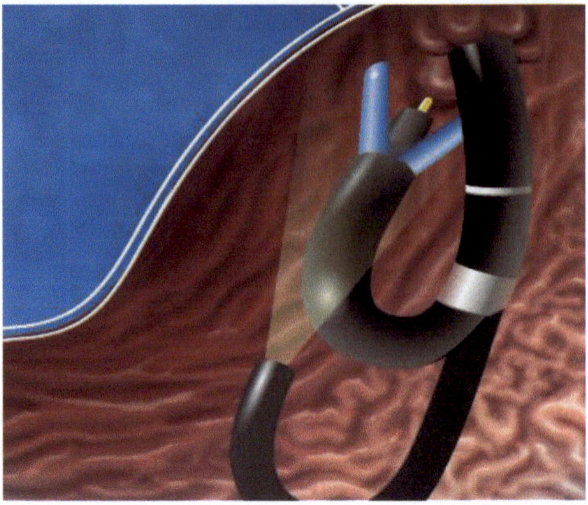

Fig. 4 Plicator® System for GERD

and "POSE" for Primary Cases"), or the Stomaphyx device. It is still under investigation. For now, it can be regarded as the most interesting contribution from the anti-reflux procedures to the bariatric field.

Anubis

Principles

The Anubis is an operative flexible endoscope created in 2005 through a close collaboration between the Team of IRCAD in Strasbourg (France) and Karl Storz-Endoskope in Tuttlingen (Germany). It was created for the NOTES procedures, permitting the access to the peritoneal cavity through the stomach as well as through the vagina and rectum. This endoscope has a diameter of 16 mm and a length of 110 mm. It is supported by two very comfortable handles and four operative channels of 2×4.2 mm and 1×3.2 mm (grasper, scissors, needle-holder, hook). Its particularity is on the tip, that has been made with the tulip flower shape in mind, permitting a small and smooth dissection of the viscera wall with the opening of its extremities; once in the peritoneal cavity, the tulip extremities are open and the operative channels appear in the clear and ready for use. It can be used not only for the NOTES procedures, but probably also for the intragastric and/or bariatric procedures, when suturing is required.

Similarities

This endoscope represents the future and the evolution of the classic operative endoscopes, because it will allow real NOTES procedures, and it is unique in its design.

Fig. 5 Anubis endoscope

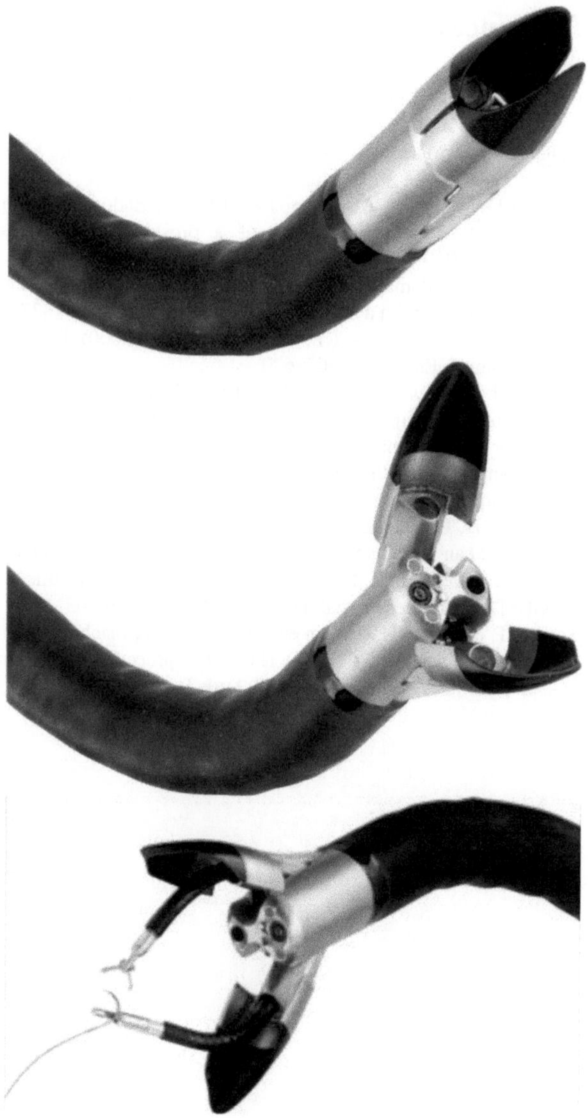

Results

Between 2005 and 2008, more than 400 experimental procedures were performed in Strasbourg on inanimate models, ex-vivo tissues, animal models and human cadavers (Dallemagne et al. 2010). The first human transvaginal cholecystectomy was performed at the end of the second year of the project (Marescaux et al. 2007). Transgastric cholecystectomy followed 6 months later, and the first five patients were successfully treated and reported with a median operative time of 150 min (range 120–180), and no intraoperative and postoperative complications (Dallemagne et al. 2009).

References

Dallemagne B, Perretta S, Allemann P et al (2009) Transgastric hybrid cholecystectomy. Br J Surg 96:1162–1166

Dallemagne B, Marescaux J (2010) The ANUBIS™ project. Minim Invasive Ther Allied Technol 19:257–261

Johnson DA, Ganz R, Aisenberg J et al (2003) Endoscopic implantation of Enteryx for GERD treatment: 12 months results of a prospective multicenter trial. Am J Gastroenterol 98:1921–1930

Marescaux J, Dallemagne B, Perretta S et al (2007) Surgery without scars: report of transluminal cholecystectomy in a human being. Arch Surg 142:823–827

Martinez-Serna T, Davis RE, Mason R et al (2000) Endoscopic valvuloplasty for GERD. Gastrointest Endosc 52:663–670

Mason RJ, Hughes M, Lehman GA et al (2002) Endoscopic augmentation of the cardia with a biocompatible injectable polymer (Enteryx) in a porcine model. Surg Endosc 16:386–391

O'Connor KW, Lehman GA (1988) Endoscopic placement of collagen at the lower oesophageal sphincter to inhibit gastroesophageal reflux: a pilot study of 10 medically intractable patients. Gastrointest Endosc 34:106–112

Oleynikov D, Oelschlager B, Dibaise J (2004) Endoscopic therapy for gastroesophageal reflux disease: can it replace antireflux surgery? Minerva Chir 59:427–435

Pleskow D, Rothstein R, Lo S et al (2004) Endoscopic full-thickness plication for the treatment of GERD: a multicenter trial. Gastrointest Endosc 59:163–171

Swain CP, Mills TN (1986) An endoscopic sewing machine. Gastrointest Endosc 32:36–38

Wolfsen HC, Richards W (2002) The Stretta procedure for the treatment of GERD: a registry of 558 patients. J Laparoendosc Adv Surg Tech A 12:395–402

B

Benchmarking of Novel Technologies in Bariatric Surgery

By Paul O'Brien: Melbourne, Australia, Centre for Obesity Research and Education (CORE), Monash University, Melbourne, Australia.

There is a huge unmet need for acceptable, effective treatments for obesity. Bariatric surgery is effective but it is largely unacceptable with only around 1 % of all potential candidates agreeing to proceed each year. We need something to offer the other 99 %. Among the factors driving people away from bariatric surgery is its invasiveness. The resurgence of bariatric surgery in the early 1990s with the introduction of the laparoscopic approach and of adjustable gastric banding showed that the less invasive the approach, the broader appeal it will have.

A new obesity procedure must be acceptable to the obese person and acceptable to their healthcare provider. Each has different needs:

Acceptable to the obese patient	Acceptable to their healthcare provider
Minimally invasive:	Low upfront cost
Endoscopic or equivalent	
Very low risk	
Minimal side effects	
Effective:	Cost-efficient and cost-effective
Good weight loss	Measure incremental cost-effectiveness ratio
Durable effect	
Co-morbidity resolution	
Adjustable	Readily reproducible
Reversible	Simple to deliver

J. Dargent, *Innovative Technologies and Non-Invasive Procedures in Bariatric Surgery*,
DOI 10.1007/978-2-8178-0404-0_2, © Springer-Verlag France 2013

We need to benchmark any endoscopic procedure against the current best practice on either side of the invasiveness gradient. Endoscopic procedural approaches to weight loss will generally fit between the relative impotence of best medical therapy and the fear of major bariatric surgery. Very low energy diets (VLED) represent the most effective of the former and LAGB represents the least fearful of the latter. These can provide current best practice norms against which to compare. We need options in between. They must be more effective than VLED. They must be less invasive and yet equally effective as LAGB.

Reasonable expectations for the comparators are as follows:

VLED	LAGB
15 kg weight loss in 3 months	30 kg weight loss over long term (>10 years)
Short term only	Less than 1 h procedure time,
No procedure at all	Outpatient – Less than 3 h length of stay
Very low cost	Low risk
Modest patient acceptability	Upfront cost US$10–15 K

For each candidate procedure we must ask: Is it safe? Is it feasible generally? Does it work? – What weight loss? What health benefit? Is the effect durable? Will patients accept it? What is the cost – in Euros, in time and effort?

Benchmark each procedure against the comparators by these criteria. Does it measure up? Can it be reasonably expected to measure up in due course? If so, go for it. Try it, measure it but be honest about it.

C

Cooperation Between the Bariatric Surgeon and the Endoscopist

Principles

The treatment of morbid obesity requires various surgical procedures, all of them being feasible through a mini-invasive approach (laparoscopy). It is highly recommended to seek and develop non invasive procedures, and thereby to redefine the cooperation between surgeons and endoscopists. Four examples of emblematic and recent techniques are picked up, two of them being surgical and laparoscopic but requesting intra-operative endoscopic control, two purely endoscopic and requesting a common approach.

Surgical Laparoscopic Greater Curve Plication (LGCP)

It competes with the laparoscopic Sleeve Gastrectomy, the gastric staple-line being replaced by two running sutures of the greater curve, thus preserved. The fact that gastric greater curve is folded into the lumen implies intra-luminal calibration, that is rendered easier through an intra-operative endoscopy.

Controlled Gastric Neuro-Stimulation (ABILITI System, Intrapace)

A trans-gastric censor is inserted through laparoscopy and connected to an electrode and a subcutaneous pacemaker, that creates a satiety effect owing to electrical

J. Dargent, *Innovative Technologies and Non-Invasive Procedures in Bariatric Surgery*,
DOI 10.1007/978-2-8178-0404-0_3, © Springer-Verlag France 2013

impulses. Preliminary tests have to be conducted via endoscopy, and the penetration of the censor has to be controlled intra-operatively.

Endoscopic Gastric Plication (POSE System, USGI Medical)

It creates a purely endoscopic selective restriction, while targeting the upper part of the fundus and the antrum. Some 15 small anchors are placed and create deep folds inside the gastric lumen. Both surgical and endoscopic skills are highly recommended in this procedure.

Hyaluronic Acid Injections at the Gastro-Esophageal Junction

HA submucosal and circular injections have been tested as a research protocol in combination or versus intra-gastric balloon (France). A moderate and temporary eating restriction takes place at the gastro-esophageal junction through endoscopy.

Conclusion

A surgery/endoscopy interaction is effectively working in most surgical procedures (gastric bypass, banding, etc.). New techniques reinforce it, and require a mutual training as well as a new distribution in the respective parts dealing with the patient.

D

Double Intra Gastric Balloon

Principles

The ReShape Duo® is a nonsurgical alternative designed for those who have exhausted their efforts with diet alone and wish to avoid, or do not qualify for surgery. It has two connected balloons, and occupies existing space in the stomach for 6 months, serving as built-in portion control, so patients feel full and satisfied with less food.

It is filled with evenly distributed 900 cc (450 cc in each balloon), 60 % more volume than typical single balloon.

Tolerability: it is designed to conform to the stomach's natural curvature for improved comfort and fewer early removals.

Safety: dual-balloon design could mitigate risk of migration and obstruction.

Placement: Under conscious sedation, the un-inflated balloons are advanced over a guidewire and precisely placed in the stomach. Each balloon is inflated with saline and independently sealed. The device is released and remains in the stomach for 6 months, serving as built in portion control.

Removal: After 6 months, the patient returns for the device to be removed through the mouth with an endoscope. Each balloon is completely drained in a controlled manner. A snare securely captures the deflated dual-balloon, and it is removed through the mouth.

Similarities

It competes with the other types of gastric balloon. If this balloon can be proven well tolerated, its design could be attractive.

J. Dargent, *Innovative Technologies and Non-Invasive Procedures in Bariatric Surgery*,
DOI 10.1007/978-2-8178-0404-0_4, © Springer-Verlag France 2013

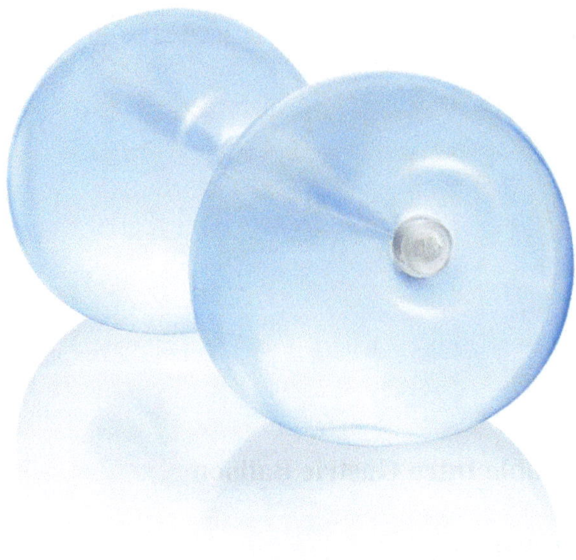

Fig. 6 Reshape intragastric balloon

Results

ReShape Duo received the CE Mark in 2007, and the medical device and its associated procedure has been refined in association with Franco Favretti and his team in Vicenza, Italy. Studies in Italy and the US have shown patients lose on average, one-third of their excess weight in 6 months.

Duodeno-Jejunal Bypass Sleeve: A Novel Approach for Type 2 Diabetes

Principles

The duodenal-jejunal bypass sleeve (DJBS), or EndoBarrier Gastrointestinal Liner® is supposed to mimick a duodenal-jejunal bypass. It has an anchor, to reversibly affix the device to the wall of the duodenum and an impermeable fluoropolymer sleeve extending 60 cm into the small bowel. The impact on diabetes mellitus caused by the foregut exclusion is theoretical: it could have a significant positive effect on glucose homeostasis in diabetic patients. Excluding the proximal intestine from nutrients by malabsorptive bariatric surgical techniques improves type 2 diabetes within days. The gut peptides Glucagon-like peptide-1 (GLP-1) and Peptide YY (PYY) are thought to play a central role in this.

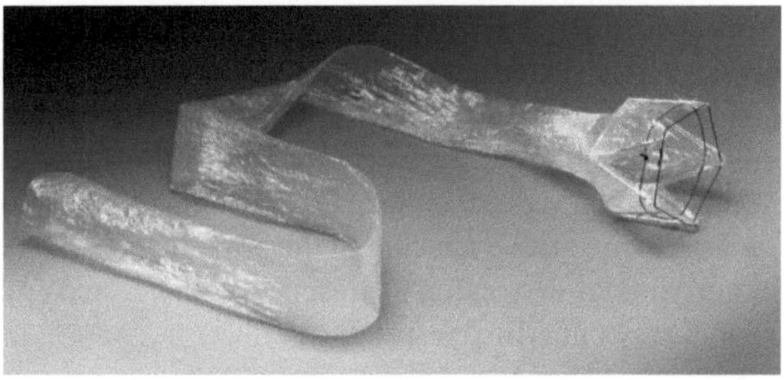

Fig. 7 Duodenal-jejunal bypass sleeve (DJBS), or EndoBarrier Gastrointestinal Liner

Similarities

Given its mechanisms of action, this procedure is meant to match the metabolic effects of a genuine gastric bypass (with a Roux-en-Y limb or with an Omega limb). Provided side-effects can be handled (anchor fixation, lumen obstruction, etc.), it could be very promising. It has similarities with other endoscopic procedures: the ValentX system provides the same tool, but with the anchors placed at the gastro-esophageal junction, suggesting a further restrictive effect.

Results

An initial study was presented by Shouten et al. (2010): Thirty patients were included in a prospective randomized trial and compared to 11 control patients. Four devices could not be placed; four had to be removed early because of sleeve obstruction (1), migration (2) and unexplained abdominal pain (1). Weight loss after 12 weeks was respectively 19 and 6.9 %. Eight patients had diabetes in the device group: six were improved and one was cured. Mean fasting glucose levels before the device placement and after 12 weeks were 11.1 and 9.3 mmol/L. HbA1c levels decreased in the same period from 8.8 to 7.7 %.

The effects of the Endobarrier® Gastrointestinal Liner on diabetes parameters and GLP-1 and PYY have been investigated by Bouvy et al. (2011): Seventeen obese T2DM patients received the EBL in combination with a low calorie diet for 24 weeks. Patients were studied prior to and 1 week after implantation, and prior to and 1 week after explantation. Blood was sampled before and 10, 20, 30, 60, 90 and 120 min after a liquid 500 kcal test meal. HbA1c, glucose, insulin, GLP-1, and PYY concentrations were measured. Results: At explantation, after 24 weeks, patients showed a mean loss of excess weight of 25.3 ± 3.0 % (mean ± SEM) while HbA1c had improved significantly from 8.4 ± 0.2 % to 7.0 ± 0.2 % ($p < 0.01$). Furthermore, anti-diabetic medication was lowered in most patients (16/17). Interestingly, within 1 week after implantation, fasting and AUC glucose concentrations were improved (11.4 ± 0.5 mmol/L vs. 8.9 ± 0.4 mmol/L and 1,999 ± 88 vs. 1,535 ± 53, both $p < 0.01$). In parallel, Area under the curve (AUC) PYY and AUC GLP-1 concentrations both increased (2,584 ± 144 vs. 4,112 ± 441 and 4,440 ± 242 vs. 6,448 ± 527, both $p < 0.01$).

Both at the time of explantation, and 1 week thereafter, the glucose parameters, fasting and AUC glucose concentrations, remained significantly decreased while the concentrations of PYY and GLP-1 had returned to normal. The observed changes in gut peptides shortly after implantation may be involved in the early improvement. These observations are in line with the hindgut hypothesis, which attributes diabetic improvement, after exclusion of the proximal small intestine, to increased secretion of gut peptides in reaction to presence of undigested nutrients in the distal gut. Other factors may underlie the sustained effect.

References

Bouvy ND, de Jonge C, Greve J et al (2011) Endobarrier r duodenal-jejunal bypass treatment results in excess weight loss and rapid improvement of diabetes in obese type 2 diabetic patients. Maastricht University Medical Centre, Netherlands. Abstract IFSO Hamburg, Sept 2011

Schouten R, Rijs CS, Bouvy ND et al (2010) A multicenter, randomized efficacy study of the EndoBarrier Gastrointestinal Liner for presurgical weight loss prior to bariatric surgery. Ann Surg 251:236–243

E

Endo-Flip System

Principles

The Endo-flip system is a tool that has been designed to measure the size and distensibility of lumens in the body using a technique called impedanceplanimetry. The first marketed application of the system is to allow the stoma of a gastric band to be set during surgery. Fluid is added the band at the end of surgery to target a stoma diameter of 6.5–7 mm. The system can be used in sleeve gastrectomy or laparoscopic greater curve plication.

Similarities

The role of stoma diameter in promoting weight loss remains controversial. Evidence suggests stoma diameter is associated with weight loss in gastric bypass procedures. In some health systems where the first band adjustment may not take place for several months after band placement, intraoperative adjustment affords the opportunity to start a patient losing weight more aggressively in the immediate aftermath of surgery, with no apparent risk, based on results published to date.

The relationship between stoma size and band fill volume varies significantly from patient to patient (Kroh et al. 2010; Snow and O'Dea 2010).

Results

Does intra-operative gastric band adjustment to a targeted stoma size improve weight loss? O'Dea J, Snow RG, Crospon Ltd., Galway Business Park, Dangan,

J. Dargent, *Innovative Technologies and Non-Invasive Procedures in Bariatric Surgery*,
DOI 10.1007/978-2-8178-0404-0_5, © Springer-Verlag France 2013

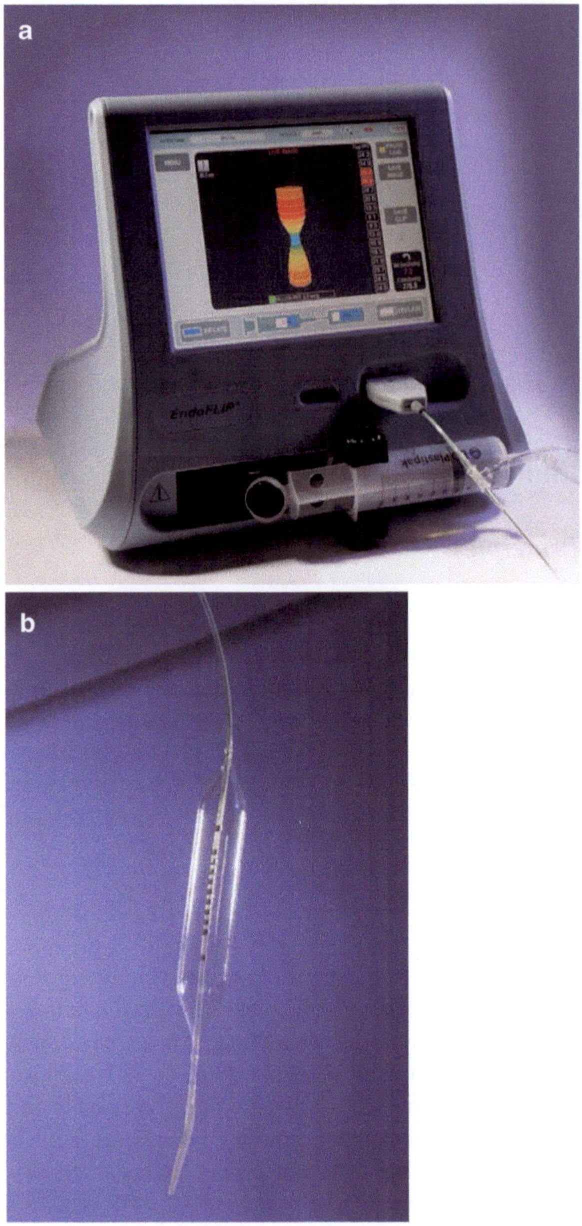

Fig. 8 (**a**) EndoFLIP System. (**b**) EndoFLIP Catheter

Galway, Ireland, National University of Ireland, Galway, Ireland, Specialty Surgery Center of Fort Worth, Hurst, TX, USA.

The authors undertook a prospective single arm clinical trial with historic controls to determine if patients could tolerate a band stoma diameter adjusted to 6.5–7 mm intra-operatively, and to assess the effect of this adjustment on post-operative weight loss, and on the number of band adjustments in the first year after

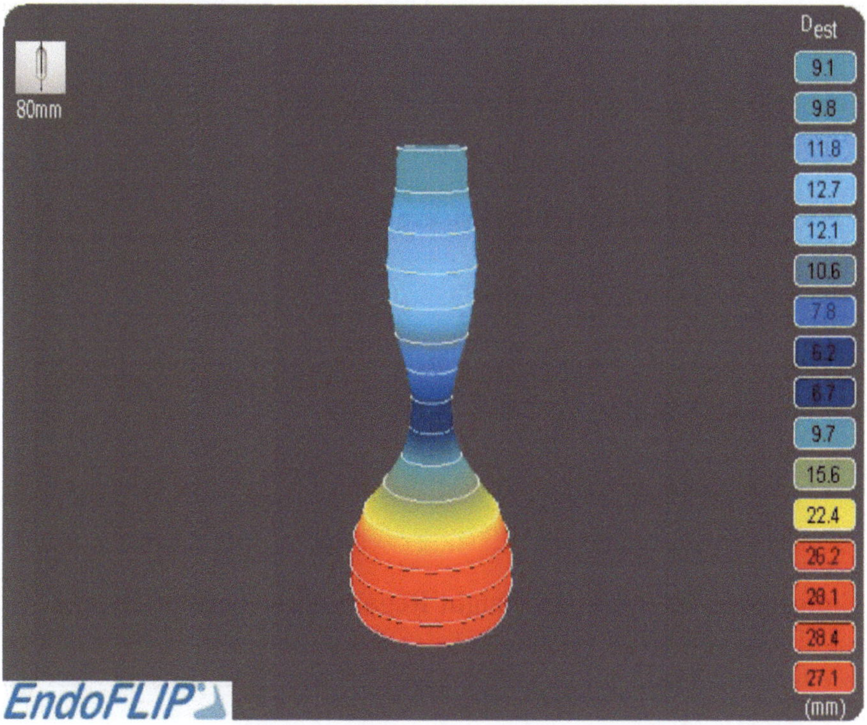

Fig. 9 Example of an EndoFLIP image when catheter is located at the centre in the band. On the right hand side, the diameter at each point along the catheter is displayed, successive diameter measurements being spaced 1 cm apart

surgery. Thirty five patients were studied, and percent excess weight loss (% EWL), as well as the number of band adjustments in the first year after surgery were compared with 49 historic controls. In the 4–6 week period after surgery, mean % EWL increases of 1.7 % (15.5 vs. 13.8 %) (p=NS) and 6.7 % (23.1 vs. 16.4 %) (p=0.06) were seen between subjects and controls for the banded patients respectively. One year after surgery, a mean % EWL increase of 11.6 % (60.3 vs. 48.7 %), p<0.05, was seen between subjects and controls for the banded patients. There was no significant difference between the average number of band adjustments, 6.5, in the 12 months after surgery, for subjects and controls. Conclusion: Intra-operative band adjustment is well tolerated. Intra-operative adjustments appeared to substantially improve early weight loss and this improvement appeared to be maintained 1 year after surgery.

Endoluminal Vacuum Therapy

(see section "Endoscopic treatment of post-op complications after gastric bypass and sleeve gastrectomy (leaks, stenosis)")

Endoscopic Re-do for Failed Gastric Bypass

(See sections "Restore Suturing system" and "Stomaphyx")

Endoscopic Re-do for Failed Sleeve Gastrectomy

(See section "RestoreSuturing system")

Endoscopic Stapling for Morbid Obesity

(see section "TOGa device")

Endoscopic Therapy for Weight Regain After Gastric Bypass

(see sections "Transport G-prox ROSE for re-do after failed gastric bypass and POSE for primary cases" and "Stomaphyx')

Endoscopic Treatment of Post-op Complications After Gastric Bypass and Sleeve Gastrectomy (Leaks, Stenosis)

Many issues can be considered, most of them dealing with general problems encountered after bypass surgery or sleeve gastrectomy, such as treatment of bleeding and/or marginal ulcer. We chose to focus on two issues, that can be treated with new options: post-op leakage and stenosis.

Stents for Staple-Line Leaks

Leaks after sleeve gastrectomy are a rare, but severe complication. Several strategies for leak repair such as stent implantation, use of fibrin glue for sealing or drainage placement and Endo VAC are described in the literature. Stents in combination with drainage can be used as a primary treatment for leakage following sleeve gastrectomy. After identifying the leak by gastroscopy different types of stents are placed covering the leak under X-ray control. Drains can be placed by laparoscopy

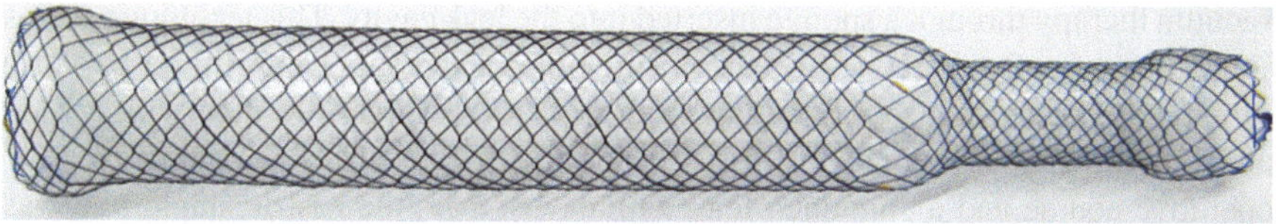

Fig. 10 Stenting a gastric leak after sleeve gastrectomy

or CT-guidance near to the leak to prevent abscess formation. A gastrograffin swallow in the follow up is used to show eventually delayed persistent leakage (e.g. due to stent dislocation or incomplete sealing by the stent). The regular time of a stent until expected remission of the leak is 6–7 weeks (unless there is a dislocation of the stent). In case of persistent leakage overlapping stent placement (Stent in Stent) to cover more distance or stent removal with application of a longer and wider stent were performed. As an adjuvant, autologous fibrin glue can be injected into chronic fistulas by gastroscopy.

Results

Stent implantation with or without autologous fibrin glue showed to be an effective treatment with a satisfying outcome (total remission rate 93 %). Stents enable oral feeding in patients with leaks following sleeve gastrectomy and help to avoid risky reoperations. A constant development in stent technology in terms of stent-material, length, form and coating may lead to a decreasing rate of dislocation and better sealing of the leakage.

Kefurt et al. (2011): Fourteen patients were treated with stents suffering from staple line leakage after sleeve gastrectomy between 2005 and 2010. A complete remission of the leakage could be reached in 64 % (n=9) after stent implantation as a single treatment. Four out of these nine patients showed a complete remission of the leakage within a regular stent residence time of 6–7 weeks. In the other five patients with persistent leakage, the stent had to be replaced 2– 4 times until complete remission. Four patients (28 %) were treated with a stent and autologous fibrin glue. One patient with no sufficient result through stenting was treated with an Endo-VAC. Dislocation and persisting leakage (fistula) were the main cause for restenting and or usage of autologous fibrin glue. Stenting alone or in combination with fibrin glue finally resulted in sealing of the leakage in 13 out of 14 patients (93 %).

Endoluminal Vacuum Therapy

In case of anastomotic leakage, lessons can be learned from non-bariatric colleagues. An innovative technique for rectal anastomotic leaks involves endoluminal vacuum therapy through a sponge inserted into the leak cavity. This technique seems simple and effective in reducing leak closure times, and could be useful for bariatric surgeons in selected cases (Kerrigan et al. 2011): A 35-year-old man with a BMI of 41 underwent revisional laparoscopic gastric bypass. He had a stormy post-operative course and a contained leak with cavity from the gastric staple line was diagnosed on contrast imaging and gastroscopy. Laparoscopy confirmed the absence of contamination in the peritoneal cavity. Initial endoscopic drainage of the leak cavity was followed by endoscopic insertion of a sponge "plug" attached to a naso-gastric tube under high vacuum pressure. Endoluminal vacuum therapy was carried out over a 7-day period with one change of sponge. Results: EVT was well tolerated by the patient. The leak cavity underwent significant reduction in exudate and wide-spread granulation tissue in-growth was rapid. The patient did not become septic at any point. After 7 days of endoluminal treatment the cavity was inspected and sprayed with fibrin glue to help prevent contagion of the leak. A further cavity was demonstrated distal to the original leak and it was decided to pursue a conventional conservative course for this. Within a week a contrast study confirmed healing of both sites with free drainage into the jejunal loop. Oral fluids were commenced with no complications. Gastroscopy before discharge demonstrated marked improvement and a further application of fibrin glue to the remnant sites was given. Total in patient stay from diagnosis of leak was 29 days. Conclusions: Endoluminal vacuum therapy for contained leaks after gastric bypass surgery is feasible and safe. It results in reduced cavity size, reduced exudate and appears to enhance granulation tissue formation. EVT could be a useful addition to the methods of managing gastric bypass leaks.

Endoluminal Over-The-Scope Clip (OTSC)

The Over-The-Scope Clip® (OTSC) is an option for the treatment of gastro-intestinal bleeding, perforations, and fistulas.

These features and therapeutic functions of the system are based on material selection and design: the superelastic Nitinol is biocompatible and, if needed, even suited and approved to be applied as a long-term implant. The dynamic tissue compression enabled by the superelastic material adapts to thickness and texture of the tissue grasped and readjusts depending to the actual requirements of the situation/tissue. This avoids over-compression and at the same time ensures constant pressure delivery to the tissue which makes it also most suitable for the treatment of chronic defects like fistulas and anastomotic leakages as well as chronic ulcers. The OTSC system is based on a transparent applicator cap and is available in a variety of different sizes and types. In addition, for precise and easy closure of even larger lesions several application aids are available: the Anchor and the Twin Grasper assist in approximating tissue in treating acute and chronic lesions. The range of application of the OTSC system includes hemostasis, closure of lesions as well as the endoscopic compression and approximation of tissue.

Treatment of Chronic Fistula

In contrast to fresh perforations the edges of an anastomotic leak and the orifice of a fistula are fibrotic. This causes problems in positioning the scope correctly at the lesion, center it right and deploy the clip. The anchor has been developed for this purpose allowing for a firm grip even on complete fibrotic tissue. Using the anchor, one has to make sure that the shaft of the instrument is well within the cap or at least level with the edge of the cap when the clip is released. It allows for a closure of the clip over the three anchor needles which afterwards can be pulled back through the clip after release. Once a clip is deployed it will stay in situ for several weeks to several months, depending on the amount and texture of the tissue secured. In most cases a surgical suture is unable to provide the same adaptability and will fail eventually. Because of its geometry the OTSC system will not impair the perfusion of the tissue and thus support better wound healing.

Clinical reports have shown promising results in the treatment of fistulas with the OTSC system (Kirschniak et al. 2011; Iacopini et al, 2010; Manta et al. 2011). The average success rate is about 80 %. Mercky et al. performed a prospective trial on patients with fistulas in the GI tract. They concluded that the OTSC system was suitable in fistulas after sleeve resection of the stomach, with a 90 % success rate. In some cases permanent closure could be achieved in a second or third OTSC system session. The clip will leave the GI tract in the grand majority of cases. Occasionally, it may be overgrown by mucosa and stay as permanent implant which is no problem because of its safety and tolerability features. Heylen et al. reported the successful treatment of weight regain due to a progressive dilation of the gastrojejunal stoma in 94 bariatric patients (over 3/4 were female) following Fobi banded bypass (Heylen et al. 2010). Best results were achieved by narrowing the pouch outlet with two OTSC system clips positioned at both angles reducing the gastric outlet by about 80 %. It is recommended to approximate mucosa and muscularis layer. For this purpose the Twin Grasper® or the Anchor are useful in order to get better control over the tissue. Heylen et al. used the spiked version of clips which provides better grip on fibrotic tissue. Due to the anatomy of the upper GI tract the preferred clip size was 11 (outer diameter diagnostic scope) and 12 (therapeutic scope). Location of clips and gastrointestinal patency were controlled by contrast swallow and by gastroscopy if clinically needed. Starting from a BMI of 45.8 (±3.6) patients had responded properly to the gastric bypass operation regarding weight loss. The average weight loss over the first 6 weeks was 4.5 kg (±2.4 kg), thereafter patients still lost 3 kg (±1.7 kg) monthly. Mean follow-up time was 12 months. No major complications occurred. A longer follow-up than is needed.

Kirschniak et al. (2011) report of a series of 50 patients that had been treated with the OTSC system for haemostasis (n=27) in the colon and the upper GI tract, closure of esophageal, gastric, and colonic perforations (n=11) as well as

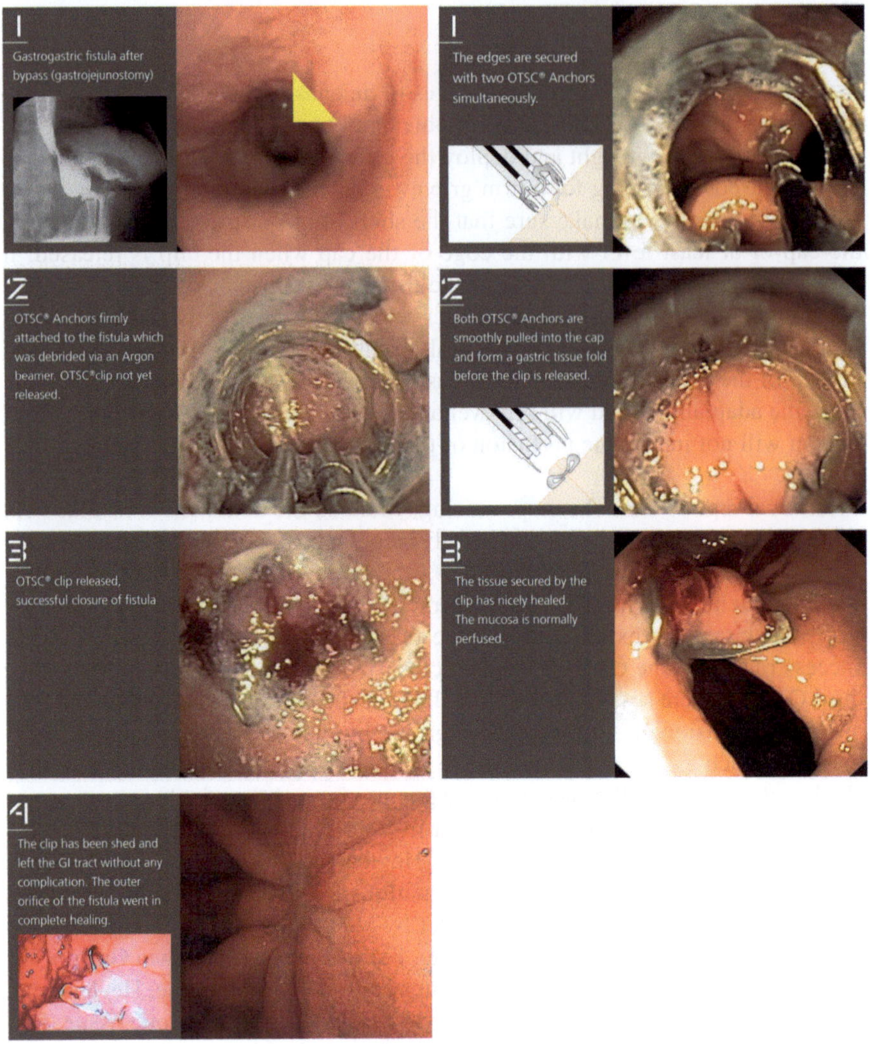

Fig. 11 OTSC system for a gastric leak

closure of fistulas (n=8) and for preoperative marking (n=4). The primary treatment was reported successful in all cases. In more detail, there were two secondary bleedings that required endoscopic re-intervention, and the permanent closure of fistulas could not be achieved in all cases. The authors conclude that the OTSC system is effective and safe for complicated bleeding and closure of fresh perforations of the gastrointestinal tract.

Treatment of Stomal Stenosis

The aetiology of stomal stenosis is multifactorial. Technical factors contributing to anastomotic strictures include the construction of the anastomosis (circular stapler), local ischaemia (reinforcement sutures, dissection, tension on the anastomosis with an antecolic, antegastric Roux limb, 21 mm staples) and a local inflammatory response (acid production, marginal ulcer, reaction to foreign material, anastomotic leak, ulceration due to ischaemia or the use of NSAIDs, alcohol or tobacco). The risk of stomal stenosis is highest in the first 2–3 months after surgery, thereafter the risk declines dramatically to negligible levels by 8–10 months. Dilatation can be achieved by fluoroscopic guided balloon dilatations with success rates of 50–60 %. Endoscopic dilatation of stomal stenosis after bariatric surgery is safe, effective and durable. It can be performed successfully by several methods including Controlled Radial Expansion (CRE) Through The Scope (TTS) balloon dilation and passage of dilators over a guide-wire (Savary–Guilliard, Eder Puestow). In bariatric surgery mainly CRE balloons have been used. Each balloon has the capability of dilating to three different sizes. Safe dilatation was at the earliest safe after 4 weeks after the operation. In patients with stomal stenosis endoscopic dilatation can be attempted in the absence of ulceration at the stoma. If there is an ulcer, patients should be placed on an ulcer treatment regime as dilatation of the stoma might cause a perforation. The initial dilation should be only enough to accommodate an endoscope of 9–10 mm for evaluation beyond to ensure that there is no ulceration distal to the stenosis, which has to heal first before resuming the dilatation. The goal stomal diameter after dilatation is 10–12 mm, up to a maximum of 15 mm. In almost no case should dilatation progress to dilators in excess of 15 mm diameter for fear of disrupting the anastomosis, resulting in leak or in progressive dilatation and loss of restrictive function. Barba et al. recommended that all the strictures had to be dilated to at least 15 mm realizing that dilating to at least 15 mm decreased the chance of symptomatic recurrence. If the scope could traverse the stricture, the latter was dilated to 18 mm. If a patient returned with recurrent symptoms and a stricture, dilation was always performed to 18 mm. This was confirmed by Ahmad et al. who mentioned that nearly 60 % of patients had complete symptomatic resolution after a single balloon dilatation session with a 15 mm balloon suggesting that this size should be used initially, and by Peifer et al., who reported a significant low rate of repeat endoscopic dilatation of strictures dilated to at least 15 mm when compared to those dilated to 12 mm or less. Most patients require a single dilatation, 5–10 % of patients may require a second dilation and a few three or more dilatations. Success rates have varied between 62.5 and 100 %. The main concerns with dilatation of the gastrojejunostomy are bleeding and perforation. Perforation of the anastomosis is related to the size of the balloon and the amount of circular force exerted on the stricture, which is related to the initial narrowing and length of the stricture. Also, the tip of the balloon can perforate the jejunal Roux limb. Perforation can also be related to the timing of the dilation after RYGBP. Schwartz et al. considered their outcomes unsatisfactory; they obtained a satisfactory result in only 62.5 % (20/32); four (12.5 %) were perforated, three out of four at the first attempt, and eight (25 %) were re-operated. The perforation rate was associated with less experience of the surgeon but might also be due to fascia lata banding present in their 1,000 RYGB patients and an overaggressive dilatation scheme. Perforations were reported infrequently by others in 1.6–3 %. An upper GI series with Gastrografin can confirm the diagnosis. Drainage of the disruption will be required. If symptoms persist, surgical revision may be required. Failure of dilatation may be predicted in the presence of torsion or angulation of the stoma and marginal ulceration with oedema.

Expectations Among Surgeons Regarding Endoluminal Therapies

Some physicians are eager to jump into new developments, some are reluctant to anything unusual and/or that has not been scrutinized and peer-reviewed. New technologies require acceptance before being launched on a large scale. Here is a useful contribution to the debate: (Brethauer et al. 2009).

Primary and revisional bariatric endoluminal procedures are currently being developed. Acceptable levels of risk and weight loss for these procedures have not yet been established. The aim of this study was to evaluate the expectations and concerns among bariatric surgeons regarding these procedures. The American Society for Metabolic and Bariatric Surgery Emerging Technologies Committee developed a questionnaire that was distributed to the membership. Risk tolerance was assessed with comparison to commonly performed endoscopic and bariatric procedures. The percentage of excess-weight loss (EWL) ranges were provided to assess the expectations for results 1 year after the procedure. Results: A total of 214 responses were returned. The acceptable level of risk to achieve 10–20 % EWL after primary and revisional procedures was equivalent to, or less than, that of a therapeutic endoscopic procedure for 81 and 76 % of respondents, respectively. The acceptable level of risk to achieve 30–40 % EWL after primary and revisional procedures was equivalent to that after laparoscopic adjustable gastric banding for 45 and 35 % of respondents, respectively and equivalent to that after laparoscopic Roux-en-Y gastric bypass for 8 and 22 %, respectively. In addition, 62 % of respondents responded that 10–30 % EWL would be acceptable for revisional procedures, and 35 % responded that 10–30 % EWL would be acceptable after a primary procedure. The primary concern was unproven efficacy, followed by durability, poor weight loss, availability of equipment, and procedural risk. Finally, 58 % would not be willing to recommend an endoluminal procedure until the efficacy has been established, regardless of the risk. Risk tolerance and weight loss expectations among bariatric surgeons are different for primary and revisional endoscopic procedures. Most surgeons were unwilling to consider endoluminal procedures for their patients until the efficacy has been proven.

Extra-Gastric Adjustable Balloon

A surgically placed external balloon has been made by the US company Vibrynt, and tested in Australia in 2010. No publication is available.

The device is implanted through a small umbilical incision, and placed in the upper left quadrant of the abdomen. It creates a smooth external compression of the stomach. Refills are allowed through a subcutaneous access.

Externally Adjustable Gastric Balloon

Principles

An intragastric balloon placed in the fundus is connected to a sub-cutaneous port, in order to allow re-fills with air. The activation of the mechano-receptors of the fundus and/or prevention of fundus expansion supposedly elicits a loss of appetite and decreases the production of ghreline. It combines endoscopy with surgery. The balloon is air-filled, and is attached to a subcutaneous port.

Similarities

Given its mechanisms of action, one may compare remotely this technique to the POSE technique that creates a partial restriction at the fundus level, in order to diminish its capability of expansion (see section "Transport G-prox "ROSE" for re-do after failed gastric bypass and "POSE" for primary cases"). It has been shown that the proximal stomach relaxes during and after ingestion of a meal, which provides the meal a reservoir: impairment of this accommodation reflex is thus associated with early satiety and weight-loss. This comparison could be more

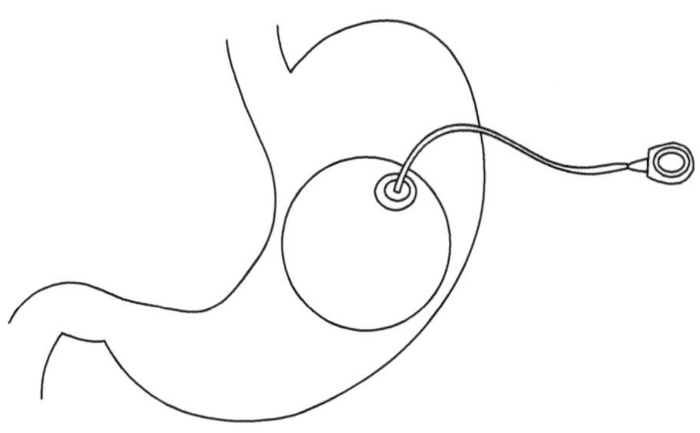

Fig. 12 Externally adjustable gastric balloon

relevant than a comparison to other types of balloons (that are purely endoscopically placed), but this remains to be further experimented.

Results

Gaggiotti et al. (2007): From November 204 to March 2007, 57 patients had ATIIP, 28M and 29F, mean age 43, 6 years (18–69), mean BMI 48.9 (33.7–81.2). Follow-up ranged from 1 to 28 months. There was no immediate vomiting. The mean volume of the prosthesis was 210 ml of air. Mean % EWL was 22.3 % at 3 months (40 patients), 28.7 % at 6 months (38) and 39.2 % at 12 months (20). A local subcutaneous infection occurred in seven cases (6.2 %), and a late infection in three (5.2 %), with port erosion.

Although potentially rare, the port-problem might be the most detrimental issue with this technique.

References

Brethauer SA, Pryor AD, Chand B et al American Society for Metabolic and Bariatric Surgery Emerging Technologies Committee (2009) Bariatric and Metabolic Institute, Cleveland Clinic, Cleveland. Surg Obes Relat Dis 5:231–236. Epub 2008 Oct 29

Gaggiotti G, Tack J, Garrido AB et al (2007) Adjustable totally implantable intragastric prosthesis (ATIIP)-Endogast for treatment of morbid obesity: one-year follow-up of a multicenter prospective clinical survey. Obes Surg 17:949–956

Heylen AM, Jacobs A, Lybeer M et al (2011) The OTSC®-clip in revisional endoscopy against weight gain after bariatric gastric bypass surgery. Obes Surg 21:1629–1633

Iacopini F, Di Lorenzo N, Altorio F et al (2010) Over-the-scope clip closure of two chronic fistulas after gastric band penetration. World J Gastroenterol 16:1665–1669

Kefurt R, Shakeri-Leidenmuehler S, Felberbauer F et al (2011) Stenting to treat leakage after sleeve gastrectomy (Medical University of Vienna, Surgery, Vienna, abstract IFSO Hamburg, September 2011)

Kerrigan D, Saha S, Magee C (2011) Endoluminal vacuum therapy (EVT)- A novel approach for contained leaks following gastric bypass (Gravitas, Liverpool, abstract IFSO Hamburg, September 2011)

Kirschniak A, Subotova N, Zieker D et al (2011) The Over-The-Scope Clip (OTSC) for the treatment of gastrointestinal bleeding, perforations, and fistulas. Surg Endosc 25(9):2901–2905. Epub 2011 Mar 18

Kroh M, Brethauer S, Duelley N et al (2010) Surgeon-performed fluoroscopy conducted simultaneously during all laparoscopic adjustable gastric band adjustments results in significant alterations in clinical decisions. Obes Surg 20:188–192

Manta R, Manno M, Bertani H et al (2011) Endoscopic treatment of gastrointestinal fistulas using an over-the-scope clip (OTSC) device: case series from a tertiary referral center. Endoscopy 43:545–548

Snow R, O'Dea J (2010) Can band fill volume predict gastric band stoma size? Gastroenterology 138(5, Supp 1):S-388

F

Flexible Endostitch

Principles

The Flexible Endostitch (Covidien®) is a device created to be placed on the gastroscope, permitting the endoluminal suturing. This device is still under development.

Similarities

This device permits the endoluminal sutures like using the RESTORe, the OESS, and the Spiderman.

Results

So far, it has been used only for experimental lab cases. It will allow the creation of the gastric restrictive compartments (similar to vertical gastroplasty or gastric banding), as well as treatment of endoluminal bleeding and fistula by suturing.

J. Dargent, *Innovative Technologies and Non-Invasive Procedures in Bariatric Surgery*,
DOI 10.1007/978-2-8178-0404-0_6, © Springer-Verlag France 2013

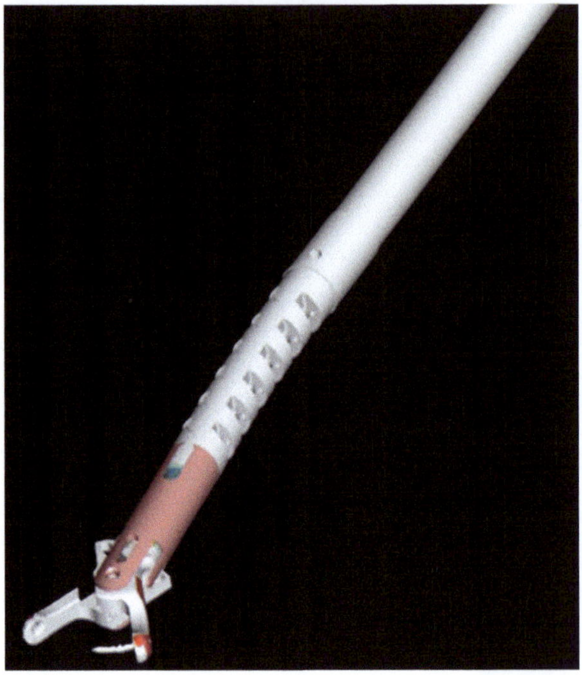

Fig. 13 Flexible Endostitch

Full Sense System for Obesity

Principles

The Full Sense® Device is a restrictive device placed at the gastro-esophageal junction, two elements supporting each other. It is more direct in activating receptors influencing weight loss, satiety, and gut hormones; it utilizes an incision-less procedure and is performed entirely endoscopically; it keeps the GI tract intact without re-arrangement; the implantation procedure is totally reversible.

Similarities

This non invasive device is supposed to match other devices described in this book, such as TOGA, gastric balloons, etc. It aims more at satiety-inducement than at restriction. Intuitively, it seems that the skills that are required are similar to the placement of an endoscopic stent (see section "Endoscopic Treatment of Post-op Complications After Gastric Bypass and Sleeve Gastrectomy (Leaks, Stenosis)").

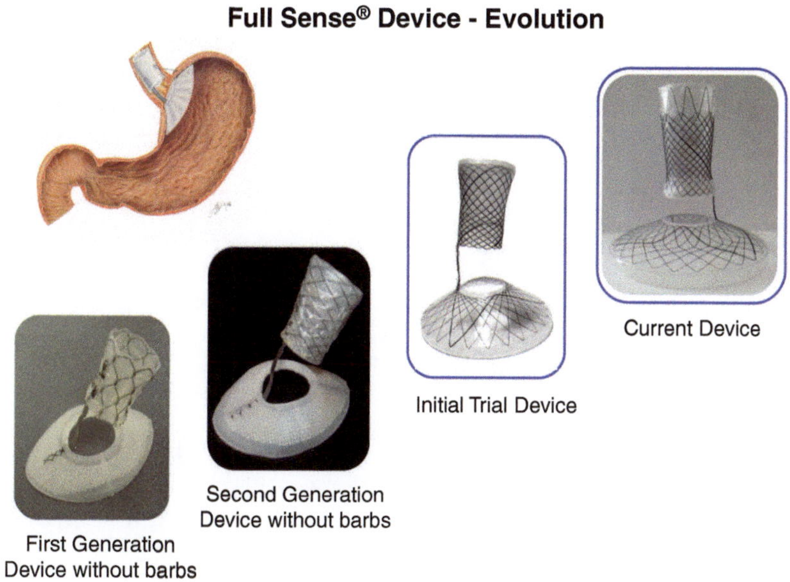

Fig. 14 Full Sense system for obesity

Results

Baker et al. Preliminary results show that 74 % EBWL has been achieved at 6 months. A randomized and blind study was implemented, in which the initial weights, interim monthly weights, and final weights were verified by an accounting firm. For the 3 month period, the average % EWL was 42 % vs the control group, and % EWL was 15.3 %. As a reminder, the BMI of the patients was 41, slightly higher than the previous study. The weight loss data achieved statistical significance at week 2 and continued throughout the study with a final p value of 0.0016.

As with all our trials, there were zero non-responders. All patients noted a marked increase in satiety. The side effect profile was favorable. The flexible implantation tool enabled most of the procedures to be performed in less than 30 min. During the 3 month formal study, none of the devices migrated into the stomach. The explants went smoothly and without complication.

The Full Sense® Device has been implanted in over 40 patients. All have experienced safe and effective weight loss, with no material side effects.

GH

Gastric Balloon

Principles

The Intragastric Balloon (IGB) is an endoscopic method to reduce weight within a short period. It is less invasive and cheaper than bariatric surgery, but can only be left in the stomach for 6 months. This is a well known procedure since the eighties, and it has been refreshed in the nineties, with a new generation of devices that have been more reliable and safer. This technique provides only a temporary weight-loss, which can be sustained further on if the proper diet counselling is not discontinued.

The overall results need to be reminded, such as in Imaz et al. 2008: Fifteen papers (3,608 patients) have been reviewed in this meta-analyzis: The mean weight-loss after balloon removal has been 14.7 kg (12.4–17), i.e. 12.2 % of initial weight (10–14.3), 5.7 BMI Unit (4.4–6.9) and 32.1 % excess-weight (26.9–37.4). Two control and randomized series have been accounted for (balloon versus placebo) with a total of 75 patients, showing a difference in weight-loss of 6.7 kg (17.6 % excess-weight loss). These two studies were thorough and double-blinded; they proved that weight-loss during the time of balloon insertion was genuine. On the other hand, there are few studies on results after balloon removal: two studies have been considered non eligible (more than 50 % of patients were lost for follow-up), and two studies have been acknowledged, with 143 patients (weight-loss at the time of removal = 15.9 kg, weight-regain during the next year = 6.3 kg, namely 39.6 % of the previous weight-loss). Even if sporadic reports have mentioned a continuation of weight-loss or weight maintenance after balloon removal, the common assumption is that weight-regain will occur to some degree during the following months, whatever diet support is provided.

J. Dargent, *Innovative Technologies and Non-Invasive Procedures in Bariatric Surgery*,
DOI 10.1007/978-2-8178-0404-0_7,

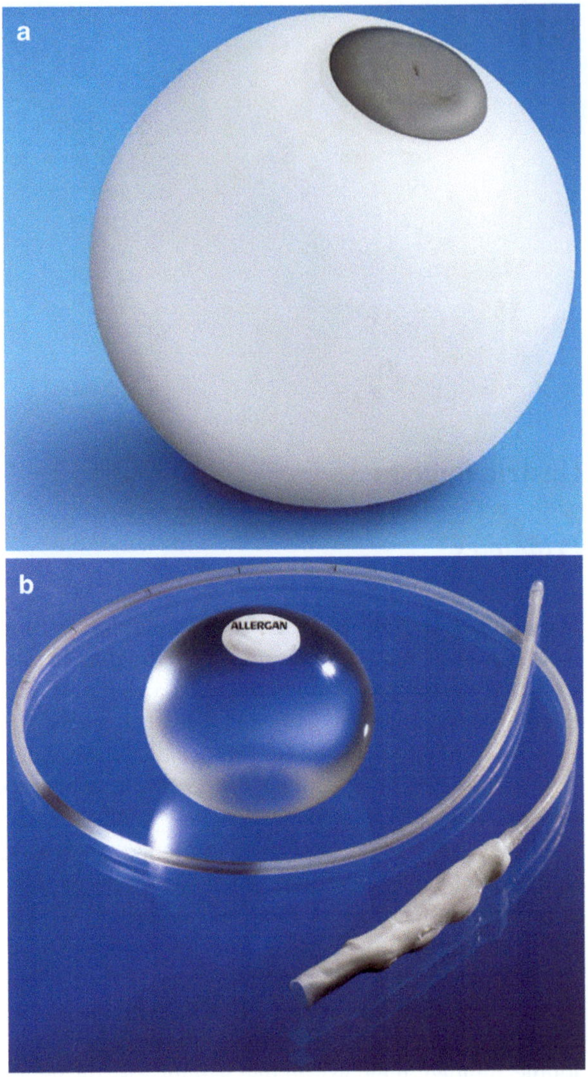

Fig. 15 (**a**) Air-filled Intra Gastric Balloon (Heliogast), (**b**) Serum-filled Intra Gastric Balloon (Allergan)

Similarities

The balloon competes with any non invasive bariatric procedure. Because of its anteriority, it provides a benchmark to any trial in this field (see section "Benchmarking of Novel Technologies in Bariatric Surgery"): not only the effect of new devices should last longer in terms of weight-maintenance, but they should also match the weight-loss that has been achieved in the studies that have been reported for 30 years.

Results

We picked up three recent papers pertaining respectively to a general and typical experience, a comparison between two balloons, and the use of the balloon as a pre-operative tool (weight-loss for any surgical procedure, or in super-obese patients before bariatric surgery), which has been for a long time the "official" recommendation of this device.

Poliwoda et al. (2011): report the results of 55 patients in Klinikum Großhadern. Methods: 24 water-filled and 31 air-filled balloons were implanted by gastroscopy. The length of therapy was 6 months. The patients were interviewed three times during therapy and also 6 and 12 months after explantation. In addition to the weight-reduction we analysed life-quality, change of lifestyle and complications. Results: Weight-loss after 6 months of therapy was 11 kg (−12 kg up to +41 kg). They could reduce their BMI by 4 kg/m^2 (−4 kg/m^2 up to +13 kg/m^2). 17 patients lost more than 15 kg during therapy (30.9 %), 8 patients lost less than 5 kg (14.5 %). The % EWL was 20 % within 6 months of treatment – the major part of weight-loss occurred within the first 3 months. IGB was more effective in patients with a higher initial weight (BMI over 40 kg/m^2), who lost 14 kg (−12 kg up to +41 kg). Patients with an initial BMI under 40 kg/m^2 lost 10 kg (−6 kg up to +35 kg). Water filled balloons seem to effect a better weight reduction (13 kg) than air filled ones (11 kg). Patients, who started physical activity (14 kg) or changed their eating habits (15 kg) could benefit more than others (7.5 kg; 4 kg). During the first 4 weeks of therapy 89 % (n = 49) of the patients complained about side effects like nausea and stomach pain. In four cases (7.2 %) severe complications occurred (erosive gastritis, perforation with peritonitis, pylorus obstruction, ulcer with acute abdomen). In three cases balloons lost volume within 180 days.

Seventeen patients underwent bariatric surgery or a second balloon treatment afterwards and continued losing weight. Long-term results are not satisfying: At the time of balloon removal the median weight of our observed group was 115 kg (71–237 kg), 12 months after treatment the median weight was 109 kg (72–165 kg) kg. During the first 6 months after therapy most of our patients lost weight, but 6–12 months after removal, most of them regained weight. Health insurance covered the cost of the treatment in 26 cases only, although 39 patients had more than two comorbidities. Conclusions: IGB treatment is an effective method to reduce weight in a short period of time. Especially in super-obese objects it can be an effective method before bariatric surgery. Long-term results without subsequent bariatric surgery are not satisfactory, because they depend on the readiness and commitment of the patients to change their life habits.

Bozkurt et al. (2011) report the results in terms of safety and efficiency using two different kind of liquid-filled balloons. Materials and methods: Fifty obese patients were prospectively divided into two groups. In the first group Bioenterics IGB (n = 25) and in the second group Silimed IGB (n = 25) were implanted endoscopically under deep-sedation anaesthesia. At the end of the 6 month period IGBs were removed. The absolute weight loss, percentage of body mass index loss (% EBMIL), % EWL, complication rates were recorded. Results: In Bioenterics IGB group there were 10M/15F, mean age 31.8 ± 12.3 years (range 16–61), mean BMI 40.6 ± 7 kg/m². In Silimed IB group there were 13M/12F with mean age 36.3 ± 10.5 years (range 17–56), mean BMI 39 ± 8 kg/m². There was no statistical difference between two groups in terms of demographics. The placement and removal of balloons in both groups were uneventful. The patients were discharged within 4 h after the procedures. No mortality or major complications were seen in both groups. Minor complications like transient nausea, vomiting (32 % vs 28 %) and pain (20 % vs 16 %) were equally seen in two groups. These minor complications were treated medically. In both groups the mean BMI went down significantly ($p < 0.001$ in both). But the absolute weight loss, % EWL and % EBMIL at the end of the treatment were statistically insignificant between the two groups (t:–0.415; p:0.680 and t:–0.239; p:0.812 and t:–0.177; p:0.860 respectively). Conclusions: Both Bioenterics IGB and Silimed IGB are equally safe and effective in weight reduction in morbidly obese patients. The Silimed IGB was found to be technically more convenient and simple.

Zerrweck et al. (2011): Super-super obesity (BMI > 60 kg/m²) increases morbimortality in bariatric surgery. We have shown previously that a significant weight-loss can be obtained in these patients with an intragastric balloon (IGB). We explored the potential benefit of preoperative IGB on the outcome of laparoscopic RYGB. Methods: We compared in a case-control study the prospectively collected records of 60 super-super obese patients (66.5 ± 3.4 kg/m²) submitted to a LGBP between 2004 and 2009, with preoperative IB (n = 23, cases) or without (n = 37, controls). Results: Baseline characteristics were homogenous in both groups. In the case group, IGB was maintained during 155 ± 62 days and induced an 11.2 ± 3.2 of % EBMIL, resulting in a lower BMI at surgery (60.5 ± 4.3 kg/m² vs 66.3 ± 6.8 kg/m² in controls; $p < 0.05$). Systolic blood pressure and GGT were also decreased after IB therapy ($p < 0.05$ vs baseline). Operative time was reduced after IGB (146 ± 47 min vs 201 ± 81 min in controls; $p < 0.01$) and mean ICU/overall hospital stay were lower than in the control group (NS). The composite end point of significant adverse outcomes (conversion, reoperation, ICU stay >2 days, overall stay >2 weeks) was significantly reduced in the IGB group (2 vs 13 in controls; $p < 0.05$). All patients were alive at 1 year and overall weight loss was similar in the case (52.4 ± 17.3 % EBMIL) and control group (50.3 ± 12.7 % EBMIL). Conclusion: Preoperative weight loss induced by IGB prior to laparoscopi RYGB in super-super obese patients was associated with a reduced operative time and a lower overall risk of significant adverse outcomes.

Gastric Balloon Without Endoscopy

Swallowing a balloon would mean that an intra-operative endoscopy is not necessary during balloon placement. This dream could come true owing to current research. Feasability studies are available and we must wait till the next edition of our directory to get results… Balloon elimination assessment could require an endoscopy or other exams though. The possibility of adding a second (and even a third) balloon has been mentioned.

Principles

Intragastric balloons have been used for weight loss with varying success. Widespread use of intragastric balloons has been limited because balloons must be placed in, and removed from the stomach endoscopically. Development of a balloon that does not require endoscopy suggests that obesity treatment with intragastric balloons has more potential. The Ullorex OIB is a large capsule that is injected with citric acid and swallowed. After 4 min, the balloon inflates to 300 cm3. Stomach acid degrades a plug on the balloon over 25–30 days, when the balloon deflates and passes in feces.

Similarities

It competes with the other types of gastric balloon. The fact that no endoscopy is necessary could be a huge advantage. A similar device is being currently tested (Obalon®)

Results

Corby et al. (2007): The purpose of this study was to test the Ullorex® oral intragastric balloon (OIB) in a sample of human participants. The Ullorex OIB was tested in 12 humans (two participants received placebo capsules). Body weight was monitored before and after balloon placement, and test meals quantified food intake among 6 of the 12 participants, all of whom received one balloon. Results: A single significant adverse event occurred. The one participant randomized to receive three balloons developed nausea and vomiting, requiring intravenous fluids, which was likely influenced by noncompliance (eating solid foods after balloon placement). Participants who received balloons had a significant mean weight loss over 2 weeks, amounting to 1.5 kg ($p<0.05$). A marginally significant food intake reduction from baseline to week 1 was found (149 kcal, 24.4 %) ($p=0.055$). Conclusions: The Ullorex OIB was successfully utilized in this study, with one serious adverse event that was likely influenced by noncompliance. Body weight and food intake data suggest that the Ullorex OIB be tested further as a possible treatment for obesity.

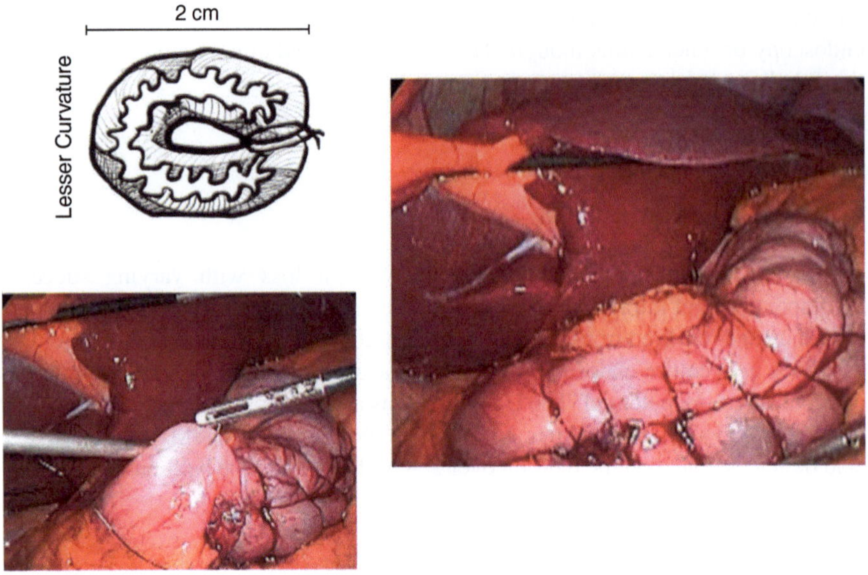

Fig. 16 Laparoscopic Greater Curve Plication

Gastric Plication (Laparoscopic Greater Curve Plication or LGCP)

Principles

Laparoscopic vertical gastric plication (LGCP) is a new surgical technique that falls into the restrictive procedure category and has gained interest in the bariatric community since a few initial studies have shown favorable results in the short term. Restrictive procedures involved the use of a foreign material, stapling devices or partial gastric resection, the LGCP surgery only involves shape modification of the stomach to achieve restriction by folding the greater curvature of the stomach inward with suture materials, thus reducing gastric capacity.

Similarities

LGCP is a strong competitor to the sleeve gastrectomy itself, although no one knows if it is likely to replace it. In this respect, the term "sleeve-killer" seems slightly exaggerated. On the other hand, LGCP could be matched by gastric internal plication (see section "Transport G-Prox "ROSE" for Re-do After Failed Gastric Bypass and "POSE" for Primary Cases") if a longer portion of the stomach could be plicated through this approach.

Results

This topic being a hot subject of controversy, we picked-up several recent and relevant papers coming either from "emerging" countries that accumulated a great amount of data (Mexico, Iran) and/or western teams commencing their experience (UK, USA, Greece).

Lapatsanis et al. (2011): From January 2009 to January 2011 a total of 155 obese patients had a restrictive bariatric procedure – 76 LGCP and 79 LSG. These patients were compared in terms of postoperative weight-loss, mean % EWL and % EBMIL. Results: In the LGCP group, mean preoperative weight and body mass index (BMI) were 115 ± 18.2 kg (range 75–161) and 40.8 ±4.5 Kg/m^2 (range 35–59) respectively. Out of 76 patients, 15 had a BMI above 45 Kg/m^2. Mean follow-up was 14 ± 2.1 months (range 6–24). The mean postoperative weight-loss was 36 Kg and the mean excess weight loss (% EWL) was 81.1 % after 12 months and 82.9 % after 24 months. The average time of follow-up was 18 months. In the group of LSG the mean postoperative % EWL was 83.7 % 1 year postoperatively and 84.9 % after 2 years. The mean % EBMIL was 81.6 %. The average time of follow-up was 18 months. Conclusions: Laparoscopic sleeve gastrectomy is a safe restrictive operation for the treatment of morbid obesity, gaining acceptance worldwide. Laparoscopic total vertical gastric plication is a valuable alternative, less expensive, with similar results, especially in patients with BMI < 45 kgr/m^2. Long-term outcomes are still required in order to evaluate the efficacy of the method, compared with other restrictive bariatric techniques.

Ortiz Lagardere et al. (2011): A total of 259 gastric plication surgeries by the same surgical team in a single bariatric center have been performed from July 2010 to March 2011, the surgical technique involved a two layered complete plication of the greater gastric curvature including anterior and posterior gastric surface, starting 1 cm from the esophageal gastric junction, ending 3–4 cm from the pylorus. Results: Of the 259 patients (Mean BMI 40.2 kg/m^2), 21 had conversions from gastric band to gastric plication surgery. Mean surgery time was 55 min, ranging from 32 to 125 min. Mortality rate was 0 %. Surgical complications occurred in eight patients (two patients with intra-abdominal bleeding that required surgical revision and blood transfusion, two cases of upper GI bleeding from ulcer formation in the plicated stomach and four cases of post operative obstructions that required redoing the plication in three patients and reversal in one). During a 3–6 months follow-up period of 118 patients (104 with no previous gastric surgery and 14 with a previous adjustable gastric band) we found a mean 42 % EWL (range 5–72 %). Out of the 118 patients, eight have undergone revision surgery to further plicate the stomach because of complete loss of restriction (six patients with previous gastric band surgery and two in the group with no previous surgery), none had complications during revision surgery. Conclusion: Although long term data on gastric plication surgery is still not available, our initial experience with this procedure has offered positive results. Additional studies and long term follow-up are needed to further define the clinical applications of this procedure.

Talebpour et al. (2011): We present 11 years experience of a new technique (vertical gastric plication), enabling us to decrease the gastric volume with long time results. History: We examined plication of different types in the sheep's stomach in 2000, then started anterior plication with voluntary patients. The details were changed three times. Methods: Three 5 mms and one 10 mm trocars are usually used. Dissection started at the greater curvature behind the pylorus and continued up to 2 cm to the angle of His. The plication went from the anterior wall of the stomach to the posterior wall (imbrication of the greater curvature inside the stomach). Nylon 2/0 was used and the bulk of each stitch was 1.5 cm, with a 1.5 cm interval. In order to preserve the fundus, deep sutures were usually added to the main row of sutures (two rows for one suture). Results: 620 patients were operated, mean age: 28 years, 500F/120M, mean BMI=42.7 (59–35), over 11 years by a single surgeon, in Tehran, Iran (2000–2011). Mean weight loss was 20 % EWL at 1 month (475), 60 % at 6 months (354), 62 % at 12 months (235), 65 % at 24 months (127), 57 % at 36 months (103) and 56 % at 48 months (75). The weight-loss curve was prominent in the first 6 months, less during the next period of time until 3 years, although the end-result was the same as other techniques. The mean time of operation was 81 min (49–152), with a discharge at 3 days on average. There were no mortality, no embolism, early intolerance. Five patients were reoperated because of a micro perforation (3), obstruction at a suture knot (1), and permanent vomiting due to adhesion between the traumatized liver and the stomach (1). The rate of weight-regain was 15 % at 4 years (11/75 cases) of operation, 30 % at 7 years (10/35) and 50 % at 10 years (5/10 cases). Conclusion: The percentage of EWL in this technique is comparable to other gastric volume restriction methods, with a limited rate of complications (mortality 0 %, reoperation 1 %, unrelated morbidity 1 %).

Narwaria et al. (2011): We aimed at comparing the surgical outcome after sleeve gastrectomy and gastric imbrication in patient with morbid obesity. Methods: This was a prospective randomized study conducted at Asian Surgicentre, Ahmedabad from September 2009 to September 2010. There were 30 patients with morbid obesity with BMI more than 35 kg/m^2. The option for surgery was chosen by randomization. The study was approved by local Independent Ethical Committee. Weight, height, and BMI of all the patients were recorded before surgery. All the associated co-morbidities with duration were recorded. The patients were followed every other month till 1 year after surgery. Results: Among 30 patients, 16 and 14 patients were operated by sleeve Gastrectomy and gastric imbrication respectively. All patients have completed 6 month follow up. 10 (33.3 %) patients have completed 1 year follow up. After 6 month mean excess weight loss in LSG and LGI was 35 % and 30 %. Mean % EBMIL was 31.1 and 24.4 % respectively. After 1 year mean excess weight loss in LSG and LGI was 49 and 45 %. Mean % EBMIL was 35.5 and 26.6 % respectively. One patient had a gastric perforation outside of the suture line and required re-laparoscopy, suture removal and closure of gastric perforation. There was no mortality. Conclusion: Both procedures are effective in reducing weight but none of them are free of complications in form of perforation and leak. Gastric Imbrication could be the best procedure for patient who wish reversion. More studies are required for long-term outcome.

Gastric Plication Associated with Banding

A gastric plication can be proposed as an adjuvant of a gastric banding (or vice and versa!). If one can be skeptical about such a combination, attention should be paid to the results of these procedures.

Huang CK promoted this combination procedure and presented it at the ***Ist NonInva meeting (Lyon, May 2011)***: The weight loss effect of laparoscopic adjustable gastric banded plication (LAGBP) was similar to sleeve gastrectomy in the early stage because of added plication effect, improving the weight loss and patient compliance. His recent case-matched study showed similar weight-loss effect up to nearly 70 % excess-weight loss and resolution of co-morbidity with sleeve gastrectomy at 2 years. It could be expected that the lower frequency of adjustment will decrease the risk of erosion and infection of the band. It combined three mechanisms, with restrictive, reductive and reversible characteristics. In the long-run, it could act to prevent weight regain after band adjustment, and can be suggested as a salvage procedure for gastric band failure.

Mozzi et al. (2011): Laparoscopic adjustable gastric banding (LAGB) is one of the most widely performed surgical procedures for morbid obesity, allowing up to 55 % of EWL. There is however a wide group of patients with EWL ranging between 25 and 50 %, where an increased effect of LAGB could be useful. Laparoscopic gastric plication (LGCP) is a new restrictive procedure that does not to require gastric resection, is reversible, and can be added to LAGB because it increases the restrictive effect while avoiding contamination of the prosthetic material. A synergistic effect may be obtained because LAGB reduces the esogastric transit, while LGCP reduces the gastric volume. Our aim was to evaluate the effect of LGCP in patients who had experienced poor weight-loss after LAGB and needed revisional surgery. Methods: 5 patients with poor weight-loss after LAGB needed revisional surgery for band slippage (2), tube disconnection in peritoneum (1), band rupture (1), isolated poor weight loss (1). They underwent LGCP in addition to band revision, in order to increase the effectiveness of LAGB. Surgical technique: two 5 mm and two 10 mm trocars were inserted, as in usual LAGB operation. After band revision, a greater curvature omentectomy was performed with the harmonic scalpel from the antrum (3–4 cm from pylorus) to the angle of His. The LGCP was then created with assistance of a 32-Ch bougie, invaginating the greater curvature with a first row of interrupted stitches of 2–0 Polypropylene. A second row of running suture of the same material was done over the whole length of the first one. Results: Postoperative course was uneventful, except slight nausea in the first few days. A gastrografin swallow on the first postoperative day showed a slow gastric transit, the band in place and the tubular shape of the plication clearly visible. The patients were discharged on the 3rd postoperative day on a liquid diet, and resumed a solid diet within 4 weeks. The mean preoperative BMI was 37.3 ± 5.19. After 3 months, while the band still was not inflated, all patients lost weight, % EWL was 18.6 ± 16.9. No symptoms of vomiting or reflux were observed. Conclusions: Surgical revisions are frequent after LAGB, in a range of 5–32 %: main causes are pouch dilatation or connecting tube complications. If band revision is needed, a % EWL lower than 50 % may be an indication to LGCP.

G-Prox for Morbid Obesity

(See section "Transport G-Prox "ROSE" for Re-do After Failed Gastric Bypass and "POSE" for Primary Cases")

References

Bozkurt S, Coskun H, Kadioglu H et al (2011) Analysis of safety and effectiveness of two different liquid-filled intragastric balloons (BIOENTERICS® VS SILIMED®). Bezmialem Vakif University Medical School, Department of Surgery, Istanbul (abstract IFSO Hamburg, Sept 2011)

Corby K. Martin, Drake E et al (2007) Safety of the Ullorex® Oral Intragastric Balloon for the Treatment of Obesity. Greenway. J Diabetes Sci Technol 1(4):574–581

Imaz I, Martinez-Cervell C, Garcia-Alvarez EE et al (2008) Safety and effectiveness of the intragastric balloon for obesity. Obes Surg 18:841–846

Lapatsanis D, Sidirokastritis G, Kontaxis V et al (2011) Evangelismos General Hospital Laparoscopic total vertical gastric plication and laparoscopic sleeve gastrectomy as restrictive procedures. Results, comparison, cost-effectiveness, differences and similarities. 4th Surgical Department, Athens (abstract IFSO Hamburg, Sept 2011)

Narwaria M, Cottam D, Sharma S (2011) Laparoscopic gastric imbrication versus sleeve gastrectomy – a prospective single blind randomized trial. Asian Surgicentre Pvt. Ltd., Bariatric and Metabolic Surgery, Ahmedabad, Salt lake City, Bariatric and Metabolic Surgery, University of Florida, Bariatric and Metabolic Surgery, Jacksonville (abstract IFSO Hamburg, Sept 2011)

Mozzi E, Lattuada E, Zappa MA et al (2011) Laparoscopic gastric plication in patients with poor outcome after adjustable gastric banding: technical feasibility and preliminary results. University of Milan, Fondazione IRCCS Cà Granda Ospedale Maggiore Policlinico, Surgery, Milan (abstract IFSO Hamburg, Sept 2011)

Ortiz Lagardere A, Martinez Gamboa A, Viramontes So M et al (2011) Initial experience with 259 cases of gastric plication surgery. Obesity Control Center, Bariatric Surgery, Tijuana (abstract IFSO Hamburg, Sept 2011)

Poliwoda EC, Lang RA, Jauch KW et al (2011) Weight reduction with gastric balloons – weight-loss, tolerance and long term results. Klinikum Großhadern LMU, Chirurgische Klinik München-Bogenhausen, München (abstract IFSO Hamburg, Sept 2011)

Talebpour M, Vahidi H, Talebpour A (2011) Eleven years experience about the new technique "Laparoscopic Vertical gastric plication" in morbid obesity, introduced for the first time in the world. TUMS, Tehran (abstract IFSO Hamburg, Sept 2011)

Zerrweck C, Maunoury V, Caiazzo R et al (2011) Preoperative weight-loss with intragastric ballon decreases the risk of significant adverse outcomes of laparoscopic gastric bypass in super-super obese patients. Lille University Hospital, Digestive and Endocrine Surgery, Lille (abstract IFSO Hamburg, Sept 2011)

IJK

Ileal Transposition

Principles

Current effective bariatric procedures such as gastric bypass generate a duodenal-jejunal exclusion, which has been implicated in the resolution of type 2 diabetes. Sleeve gastrectomy could be combined with ileal transposition (SGIT), in order to be as effective as Roux-en-Y gastric bypass (RYGB) to induce glucose control. This operation is not yet evaluated in humans, although it has been reported.

Similarities

Ileal transposition is supposed to compete with other metabolic operations, providing a long-lasting effect on glycaemia for instance.

Results

Boza et al. (2011): Current effective bariatric procedures such as gastric bypass generate a duodenal-jejunal exclusion, which has been implicated in the resolution of type 2 diabetes. The aim of this study was to test the hypothesis that sleeve gastrectomy with ileal transposition (SGIT), a new procedure, is as effective as Roux-en-Y gastric bypass (RYGB) to induce glucose control on an obese rat model of type 2 diabetes mellitus. Methods: Twenty eight obese diabetic Zucker rats, weighing 571 ± 151 g were assigned into three procedures: SGIT (n = 11), RYGB (n = 7), and sham operation (n = 10). Animals were followed, evaluating weekly weight

J. Dargent, *Innovative Technologies and Non-Invasive Procedures in Bariatric Surgery*,
DOI 10.1007/978-2-8178-0404-0_8, © Springer-Verlag France 2013

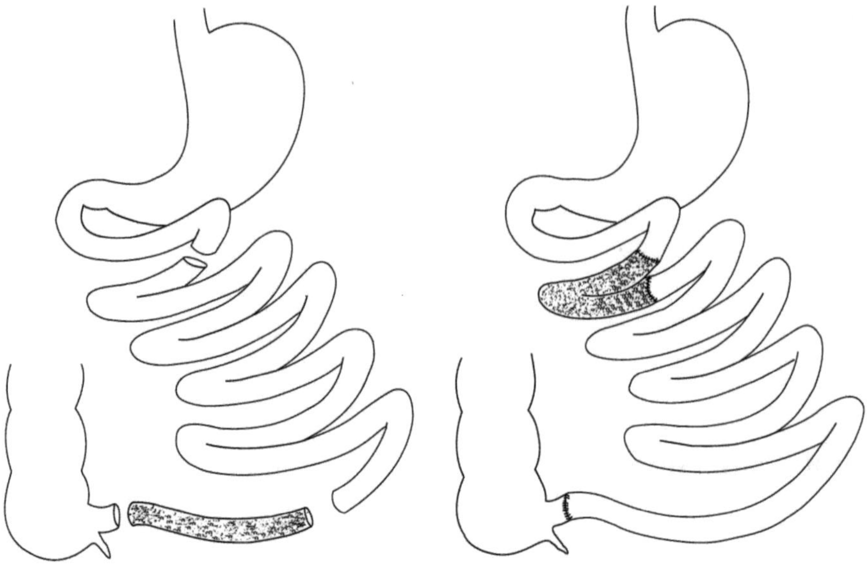

Fig. 17 Ileal Transposition

increase and food intake. We performed an insulin tolerance test after 8 weeks and measured serum peptide tyrosine-tyrosine (PYY 3–36) and ghrelin levels.

Results: 9 weeks after surgery, sham-operated animals increased their body weight by 24 %. In far contrast, SGIT and RYGB rats weighed 21 and 18 % less than sham animals, respectively (sham, 884 ± 15 g; SGIT, 720 ± 19 g; RYGB, 754 ± 14 g; $p<0.001$). No significant differences were found between SGIT and RYGB. Cumulative food intake in SGIT and RYGB procedures decreased by 29.6 and 32.9 %, respectively (sham, 576.3 ± 33 g; SGIT, 405.8 ± 10 g; RYGB, 386.4 ± 21 g; $p<0.001$). No differences were found between SGIT and RYGB rats. Sixty minutes after oral gavage, PYY levels were increased by 185 and 74 % in SGIT and RYGB, respectively (sham, 63.4 ± 2.1 pg/ml; SGIT, 192.7 ± 17 pg/ml; RYGB, 117.7 ± 4.8 pg/ml; $p<0.001$). Glucose tolerance was improved after SGIT and RYGB surgery demonstrated by area under the curve analysis (sham, 27,090 ± 1,424; SGIT, 17,704 ± 1,288 mg/dl; $p<0.018$; RYGB, 16,212 ± 2,522; $p<0.01$). Conclusion: SGIT proved to be as effective as RYGB on obese diabetic rats as a weight loss procedure. Also, glucose homeostasis improved in SGIT, similar to RYGB, in spite of the absence of duodenal-jejunal exclusion. This observation does not support the theory that RYGB reversal of diabetes is due to duodenal-jejunal exclusion.

Injection at the GE Junction

Principles

In order to gain more acceptance, research for non invasive techniques is mandatory in the field of bariatric surgery. A preliminary useful step is the combination of these

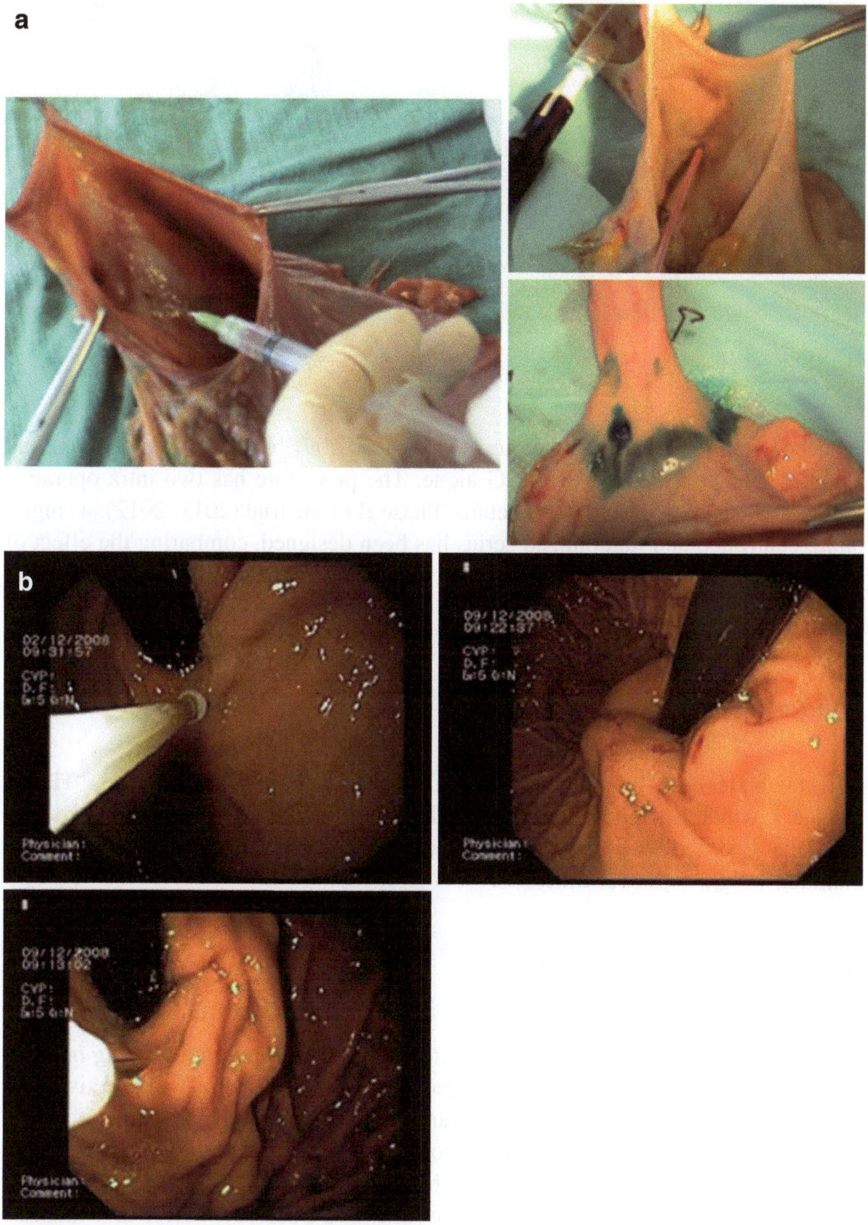

Fig. 18 (**a**) Injection at the GE junction (cadaver study); methylene blue injection matches the position of a gastric band. (**b**) HA injection at the gastro-esophageal junction, endoscopic view (retrovision). (**c**) Study protocol: HA injection followed by intra gastric balloon insertion

techniques with current mini-invasive procedures that need further evaluation. We suggested that sleeve gastrectomy (SG) can be associated with a sub-GE junction injection of hyaluronic acid (HA). Hyaluronic acid is currently used in cosmetic surgery; the device we implanted is also used for knee arthritis. Four patients have

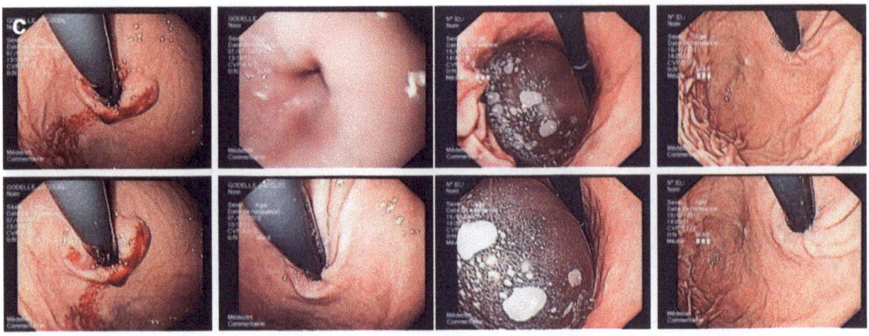

Fig. 18 (continued)

been operated on a 3 months period (11/08 to 01/09) by SG+HA injection, and matched with four patients with SG alone. The procedure has two intra-operative stages, and has been described in details. Phase II of the trial (2011–2012): a single-blind, controlled and randomized series has been designed, comparing the effect of HA injection and intragastric balloon, and testing the combination of both techniques.

Similarities

This methods bears comparison with the TERIS device (see section "TERIS Device"), which is supposedly long-standing, whereas HA is a temporary product. It has therefore the potential to be combined with other bariatric methods that fail to maintain weight-loss over time.

Results

The preliminary results have been presented at ***the IInd Non-Inva meeting in Lyon (April 2012) by J Dargent***: Ninety-one patients were included in a prospective controlled study in single-blind, and were randomly assigned to three groups: group 1 had a stand-alone balloon (Allergan®), group 2 had a balloon, followed by HA injection at removal time (6 months), group 3 had an HA injection followed by a balloon 6 months afterwards. Mean BMI at baseline was 33.8 (27–43.7); at 6 months (N=54) % EWL in group 1, 2 and 3 was respectively 18.6, 33 and 18.6; at 12 months (N=21) 18.8, 30.8, 31,6; at 18 months (N=12) 16.6, 37,2, 37.9. Eighteen months is the key-period of time since we know from the literature that weight-regain after balloon removal amounts to 40 % within 1 year. The results are encouraging, and further studies are to be implemented. So far, group 3 seems intuitively the most interesting, i.e. HA injection followed by balloon placement between 2 and 6 months afterwards seems the most relevant strategy, although this entails three anaesthesia.

Intra Gastric Injection of Botulinum Toxin

Botulinum toxin A (BTX-A) is a powerful and long-acting inhibitor of muscular contractions in both striated and smooth muscles. Hypothetically, it should inhibit the acetylcholine-mediated perilstalsis, which is mainly responsible for gastric motility, and thereby induces slowed gastric emptying, early satiety and weight-loss.

Mittermaier et al. (2007): After approval by the University Ethic Committee, 10 F patients with class I obesity (BMI 30–35) were double-blind randomized into two groups (BTX-A and 0,9 % saline). In group 1, 200 u BTX-A were injected endoscopically into the antrum and the distal gastric body. In group 2, 0.9 % saline was injected endoscopically in the same places. Body-weight and feeling of satiety were recorded monthly over a period of 6 months. Results: Both groups showed no significant weight reduction ($p>0.05$). One patient in group 1 and 2 patients in group 2 reported a feeling of early satiety. No adverse effects were observed. Conclusion: Intragastric injection of BTX-A for the treatment of obesity does not seem to reduce body weight.

Intra Gastric Injection of Satiety-Hormone-Producing Cells

Alverdy et al. (2008): Repopulating the foregut mucosa with epithelial cells that release an anorexigenic quantity of gut-derived satiety hormones in response to food has the potential to offer a physiologic approach to treating obesity. Reseeding of the foregut mucosa (stomach, duodenum, and proximal jejunum) with cultured cells programmed to release increased amounts of satiety hormones such as peptide YY or GLP-1 could be accomplished by injecting cultured peptide-producing epithelial cells directly into the intestinal submucosa. Implanted cells could be fused with fluorescent probes that allow for their endoscopic detection and hence excision or replacement in the event that the response becomes excessive or diminished. We have proved the feasibility of this approach by implanting pancreatic cells into the stomach submucosa of rats and demonstrated that cells are viable 7 days after implantation. Once stem cells lines that differentiate to peptide YY or GLP-1 cells are developed, they could be easily implanted endoscopically.

Internally Adjustable Gastric Balloon

Principles

The objectives of this kind of balloon are to prevent four major drawbacks of the current intragastric balloons: intolerance in the early period; insufficient weight loss after 3 months; risk of bowel obstruction, which entails its removal at 6 months; the need for a dedicated extraction tool.

The introduction of an adjustable balloon could improve comfort and offer greater efficacy. A migration prevention function, safely enabling prolonged implantation, could improve efficacy and weight maintenance post extraction. Polypectomy snare extraction would also be beneficial.

The first implantations of an adjustable balloon with attached migration-prevention anchor have been reported with the Spatz® Adjustable Balloon, which is mounted on a curled non-crushable catheter that straightens over a guidewire, and passed transorally, under conscious sedation. The non-crushability of the catheter loops is mediated by an internal chain. Post-implantation, an extractable inflation tube housed in the catheter can be snared endoscopically and pulled outside the mouth for volume adjustments.

The latest generation Spatz balloon incorporates a completely closed catheter loop to improve its anti-migration function. The loop unlocks endoscopically at the end of the 1 year implantation; a kink resistant inflation tube enables easier inflation and deflation.

Similarities

This internal adjustability matches more or less the external adjustability described with the previous balloon. The Allergan® balloon had this opportunity as well, through its own valve, but it has been actually seldom used.

Results

Machytka et al. (2011): Eighteen patients (15 female, 3 male) had the procedure, with mean BMI 39,4 (range 29.4–53.2) and mean weight 114.9 kg (range 73,5–163 kg). They had a mean balloon volume of 406.9 cc (range 350–600 cc) of saline. Results: Mean weight loss at 24 weeks was 15.6 kg with a 26.4 % of % EWL, and 35.5 kg with a 67.3 % EWL at 52 weeks. Sixteen adjustments were successfully performed. Six downward adjustments alleviated intolerance, yielding an additional mean weight loss of 4.6 kg. Ten upward adjustments for weight loss plateau yielded a mean additional weight loss of 8.1 kg. There were no major complications, however, seven of the 18 balloons were removed. Conclusion: The Spatz ABS has been successfully implanted in eighteen patients. Upward adjustments yielded additional weight loss. Downward adjustments alleviated intolerance, with continued weight loss. Eight extractions were performed with a polypectomy snare. Preliminary 1 year results are encouraging.

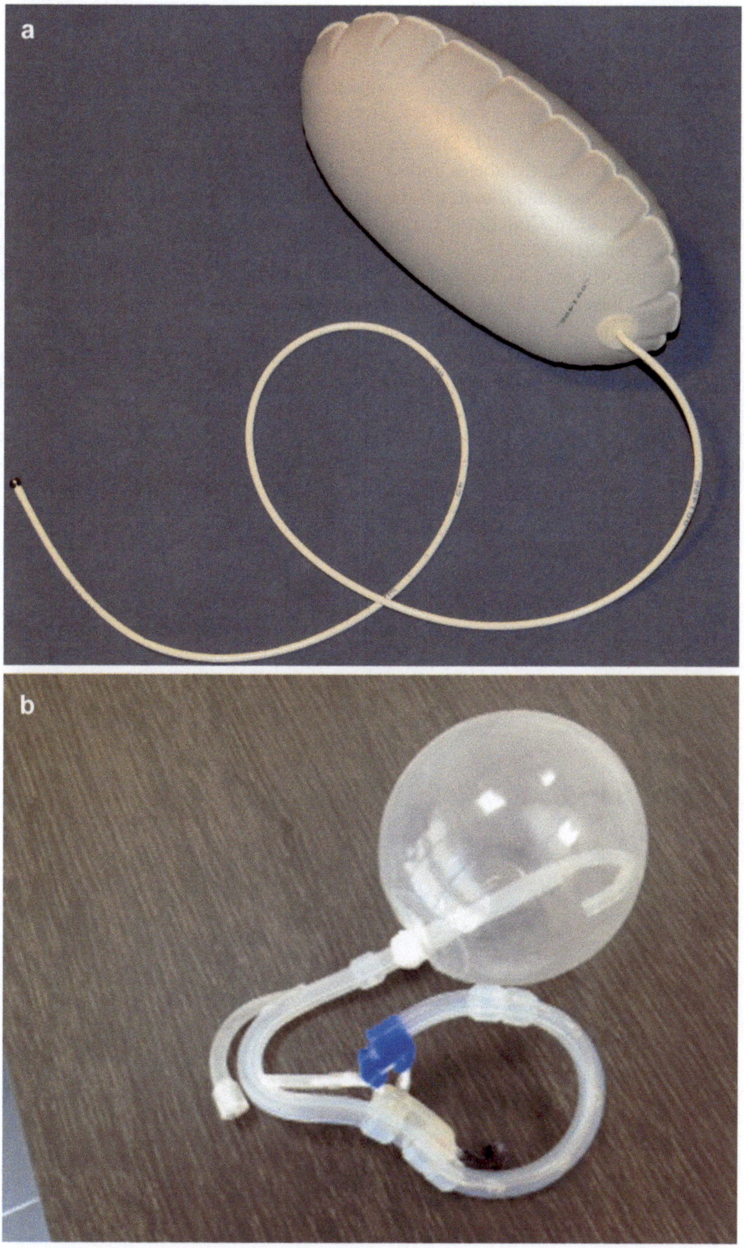

Fig. 19 Internally adjustable gastric balloon (**a**) LPE Balloon (**b**) Spatz Balloon

References

Alverdy JC, Prachand V, Flanagan B et al (2009) Bariatric surgery: a history of empiricism, a future in science. J Gastrointest Surg 13(3):465–477. Epub 2008 Nov 13

Boza C, Muñoz R, Yung E et al (2011) Sleeve gastrectomy with ileal transposition (SGIT) induces a significant weight loss and diabetes improvement without exclusion of the proximal intestine. Division of Laparoscopic and Bariatric Surgery, Department of Surgery, NewYork-Presbyterian Hospital, Weill Medical College of Cornell University, New York. J Gastrointest Surg 15 (6):928–934. Epub 2011 Mar 24

Machytka E, Mathus-Vliegen EM, Gostout CJ et al (2011) A Novel Adjustable Intragastric Balloon (IGB) to treat Obesity: A Pilot Stud. University of Ostrava, Faculty of Medicine, Czech Republic, Academic Medical Centre, Amsterdam, Mayo Clinic, Rochester, Tufts Medical Center, Surgery and Bariatric Surgery, Boston, United States, University of Medicine and Dentistry, Camden, Mt. Sinai Hospital, New York, Assuta Hospital, Tel Aviv (abstract IFSO 2011, Hamburg)

Mittermaier R, Keller C, Geibel J (2007) Intragastric injection of botulinum toxin a for the treatment of obesity. Obes Surg 17:732–736

L

Laparoscopic Gastric Plication

(see section "Gastric Plication")

Laparoscopic Instruments for Gastric Plication

Instead of running sutures, a specific instrumentation has been developed by Ethicon® in order to facilitate the surgical plication. The device is under trial and not available.

Likewise, one has suggested the use of a dedicated balloon to calibrate the residual gastric pouch after plication (see section "MID-Sleeve").

Laparoscopic Micro-Instrumentation

Principles

Micro-instrumentation, most often consisting in 3 mm access, minimizes the surgical access and competes with the single trocar (or single incision) approach. The herein described instrument makes it possible to combine this concept with real 5 or 10 mm instruments, thereby providing a match to the usual specifics of a given bariatric procedure.

J. Dargent, *Innovative Technologies and Non-Invasive Procedures in Bariatric Surgery*,
DOI 10.1007/978-2-8178-0404-0_9, © Springer-Verlag France 2013

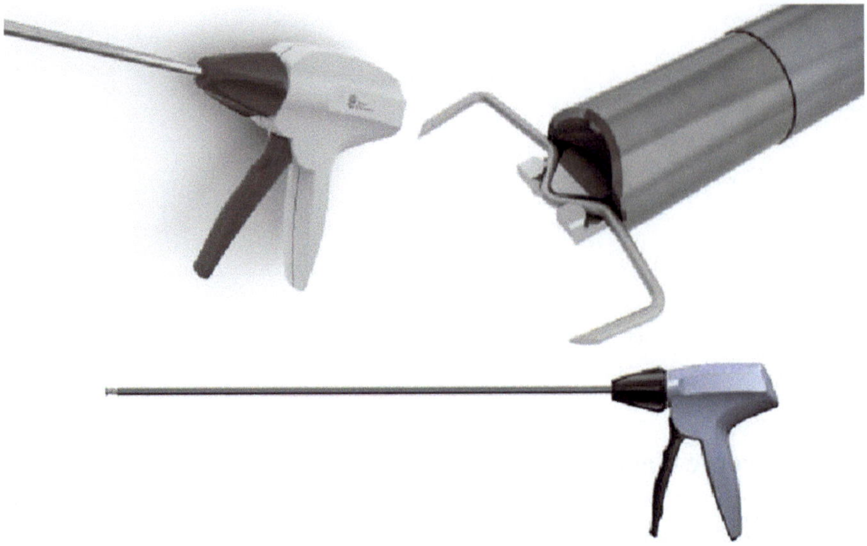

Fig. 20 Laparoscopic instruments for greater curve plication

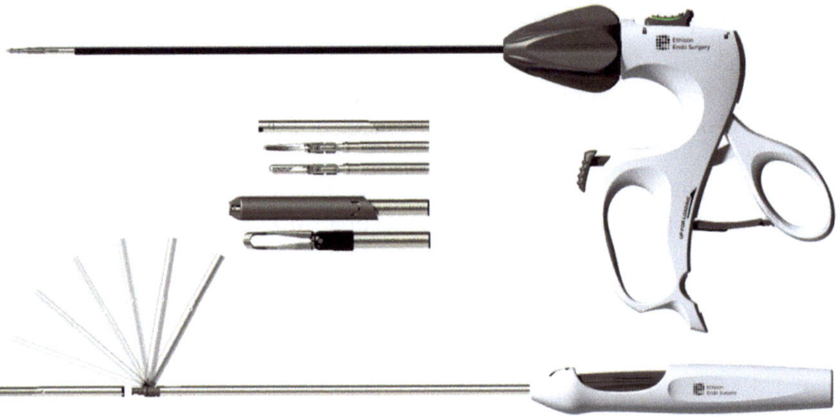

Fig. 21 PSS micro-instrumentation

An Original Device

The PSS (Percutaneous Surgical Set) is a sterile, single patient use system offering a series of 5 or 10 mm tool attachments that are loaded onto a 3 mm percutaneous shaft, meaning it's inserted into the body like a needle instead of through a trocar, thereby reducing tissue trauma.The device's handle has a 3 mm shaft with a pointed obturator tip that is used to gain entry into the patient percutaneously (without a trocar). Once the shaft is through the patient's body wall, three larger tool attachments (a 5 mm grasper, 5 mm Maryland dissector and a 10 mm Babcock) are inserted through a trocar and quickly assembled in situ with the help of the loader. This allows the surgeon to reduce the incision size but still provides the trusted 5 or 10 mm tool attachments.

The PSS provides several significant benefits: (1) Less tissue trauma – On average, the tissue defect resulting from the PSS is five times smaller than the defect from a 5 mm trocar (Pre-clinical study). This can potentially eliminate the need to surgically close the incision site, and can potentially lead to less pain and a better aesthetic outcome for the patient. (2) Better access – Because its tissue defect is so minimal, the PSS can be repositioned (removed from one incision point and moved to another) to enable the optimal angle and reach on the targeted tissue. (3) Same trusted performance – The PSS enables performance similar to trusted 5 or 10 mm instruments. PSS offers the full sized 5 or 10 mm tool attachments.

M

Magnetic Internal Video

Principles

Placement of multiple trocars is a standard technique in most laparoscopic bariatric procedures. Wound healing, portal hernia and cosmetic results can lead to complications in this kind of surgery. Single port procedures seem to give better results but technical challenges and limited working space are major limitations. Through the cooperation of surgeons and robotic engineers, a magnetic remotely controllable video-endoscopic capsule device dedicated to mini-invasive surgery has been developed.

Similarities

MIM camera was thought to allow a less number of incisions required for minimal invasive surgery, to improve the angle view to 360°, and to facilitate the instrument's triangulation, thanks to the use of multiple devices for vision and lighting. It is clearly competing with other minimally invasive approaches such as SILS or micro-instruments.

Results

Di Lorenzo et al. (2011): The aim of the study is to prove the feasibility and safety of using MIM (Magnetic Internal Mechanism) capsule instead of a standard laparoscope to carry out a laparoscopic procedure in vivo animal trial. Material and methods: The trial has been carried on using two MIMs and two illuminating bars with a

J. Dargent, *Innovative Technologies and Non-Invasive Procedures in Bariatric Surgery*,
DOI 10.1007/978-2-8178-0404-0_10, © Springer-Verlag France 2013

diameter of 12 mm and a length of 40 mm. As a first trial, after the placement of a trocar, a standard laparoscope has been inserted to perform a previous examination of the abdominal cavity and to obtain a record of the experiment from another point of view. We introduced laparoscopic instruments and MIM capsules through two dedicated trocars. The prototype was provided of a wire for experimental purposes although wireless technology has already been proven feasible for power supply and image transmission. Two intracapsular moveable permanent magnets allow fine positioning, and an externally applied magnetic field permits movement and stabilization of the cameras. Results: We carried out successfully laparoscopic procedures including cholecystectomy and a gastric bypass. MIM cameras and on-board illumination system was adequate to provide good imagery of nearby abdominal structures. A great advantage was obtained from the use of different cameras placed in different site of the abdominal cavity. Fine control of capsule navigation and rotation was achieved during the whole procedure. Precise camera steering and full 360° viewing was possible. Conclusions: This preliminary study demonstrated the feasibility of a laparoscopic procedure carried out using MIM capsule. Most of complications of single port surgery would be solved inserting multiple MIM devices through the same trocar. The presence of multiple video capsules enabled a complementary view of the structures by many angles of sight. This is particularly useful in obese patients where abdominal fat can negatively impact on vision in abdominal recesses. The use of this device can also reduce the conflict in the abdominal cavity between laparoscopic instruments allowing a better triangulation. More trials have to be performed but MIM system would potentially become a feasible option for single port and natural orifice transluminal endoscopic surgery (NOTES).

MID-Sleeve

The MID-Sleeve® is a silicone tube 12.5 mm in diameter (36 F) with a balloon at its distal end. The shape of this balloon is designed to fit into the gastric antrum, allowing accurate and repeatable calibration. It has been specifically design to improve the performance of the sleeve gastrectomy, because it can foretell the exact volume of the stomach remnant after the gastrectomy. It can also be used as a suction system to remove air or liquid during the procedure.

If one deems that the most important post-op issue with laparoscopic vertical plication (see section "Laparoscopic Greater Curve Plication") is gastric emptying and the tightening of the antrum (creating excessive vomiting), then calibrating the antrum with the Mid-sleeve could be valuable. Prospective trials have to be carried out.

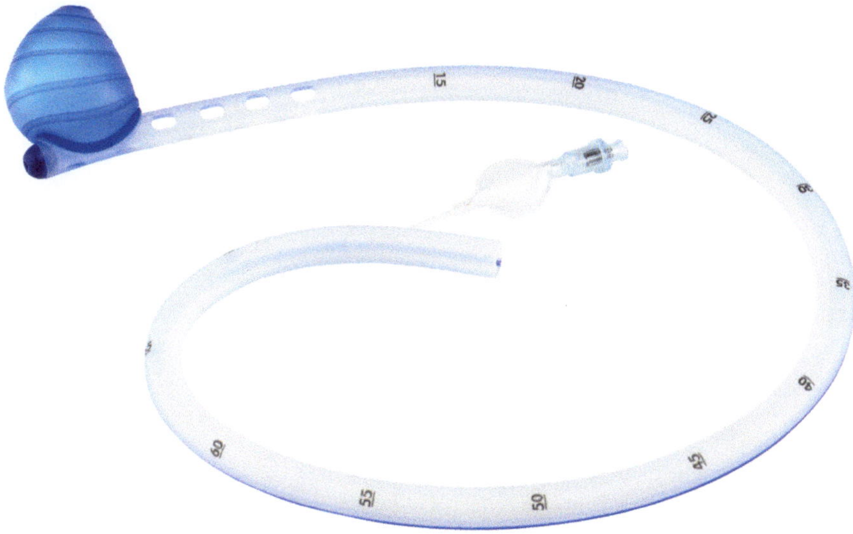

Fig. 22 MID-Sleeve

Reference

Di Lorenzo N, Arcudi C, Divizia A et al (2011) A camera integrated in a magnetic internal mechanism (MIM) for single access laparoscopy: application in bariatric surgery. Università di Roma Tor Vergata, Department of Surgical Sciences, Roma, Scuola Superiore Sant'Anna, Department of Biomedical Robotics, Pisa (abstract IFSO Hamburg, Sept 2011)

N

Neuromodulation in Obesity Treatments

Principles

Shikora (2011): Neuromodulation represents a group of new surgical approaches to the treatment of obesity and associated metabolic disorders that involves the application of a small patterned electrical impulse to a target organ. The target organ may include the stomach, duodenum, small intestine, vagus nerves, the adrenal glands, or the brain. Changing the pattern and amount of energy delivered can also alter the desired effect. The impulse can augment or modify normal physiologic responses or block them. There is a growing body of research to suggest that the technology is safe. In addition, at least some of the neuromodulatory technologies have the potential to provide beneficial weight loss and positive effects on the associated metabolic conditions. Methods: This presentation will review and analyze the latest published research evaluating neuromodulation. Results: To date, the published data with neuromodulation suggests that there may be potential for benefit with some of these technologies. Thus far, promising results have been reported in small open label trials with short follow up. The few large prospective, randomized, blinded trials have not yet demonstrated clinically relevant efficacy. Conclusion: Neuromodulation offers safe and less complex options to the conventional surgical approaches to morbid obesity. However, the early data does not support its clinical application. More study would be required before the technology is deemed efficacious.

Three systems are currently competing and are reported here. Two of them (ABILITI and TANTALUS) deal with a satiety-inducing stimulation that is more or less monitored through gastric distension measurement, thus allowing a theoretical fine-tuning of electrical stimulation. The third one (V-BLOC) aims at direct vagal stimulation, which has been suspected for a long-time of being instrumental in decreasing hunger and enhancing satiety (as well as vagotomy). Trials are being

J. Dargent, *Innovative Technologies and Non-Invasive Procedures in Bariatric Surgery*,
DOI 10.1007/978-2-8178-0404-0_11,

conducted with each of these devices, some of them focusing more specifically on comorbidities such as type 2 diabetes.

ABILITI System

Seyfried et al. (2011): Alterations of eating behavior in obese subjects treated with the abiliti® System (IntraPace, Inc.) were assessed in an ongoing prospective clinical multicenter trial. The ability® system is a closed loop gastric electrical stimulation device which features a transgastric sensor to detect food intake and an accelerometer to record physical activity. The stimulator delivers a tailored gastric stimulation in response to food consumption, aiming to induce early satiety. Methods: The abiliti® system was implanted laparoscopically. The subjects were seen regularly for weight measurement, review of food intake, activity data and stimulation regimen adaptation. Subjects completed a validated three factors eating questionnaire (TFEQ) before, 3 and 6 months after therapy activation. The questionnaire assesses the cognitive restraint (factor 1), which has been shown to be associated with successful treatment of obesity, the loss of control (factor 2) which increases the probability of relapse, and hunger (factor 3). The analysis compared the three factor scores obtained at 3 and 6 months to the baseline scores. Results: Thirty-four obese subjects (BMI 35–55 kg/m^2) underwent successful device implantation. Twenty-seven subjects completed the 6 months follow up. Thirty three subjects reached 3 months therapy with a mean % EBWL of 15.9 % (±9.3) and a mean total weight loss of 7.2 kg (±4.0). Twenty seven subjects reached 6 months therapy with a mean % EBWL of 23 % (±11.7) and a mean total weight loss of 10 kg (±5.5). l TFEQ performed at 3 months showed a significant increase of factor 1 and a significant decrease of the factor 2 and factor 3 compared to baseline (paired t-test $p<0.001$). The decrease of the factor 2 and factor 3 persisted at 6 months (paired t-test $p<0.001$). Conclusion: Preliminary results of gastric electrical stimulation using the Abiliti® system in obese subjects demonstrate that the therapy is well tolerated and leads to significant weight loss. We suggest that weight-loss is achieved due to the assessed alteration of eating behavior in particular the reduction of loss of control and hunger.

TANTALUS System

Bohdjalian A and Tantalus Research Group (2011): The majority of T2DM patients cannot be managed by medication alone, thus, metabolic surgery as a treatment for T2DM is becoming more acceptable. However, it is considered as a major intervention with significant drawbacks and side effects. The TANTALUS System®, a meal initiated GI stimulator, is implanted in T2DM obese patients using a reversible laparoscopic procedure. The risk-benefit profile of this System was previously demonstrated, however, it was limited to a short period follow up. We present here longer

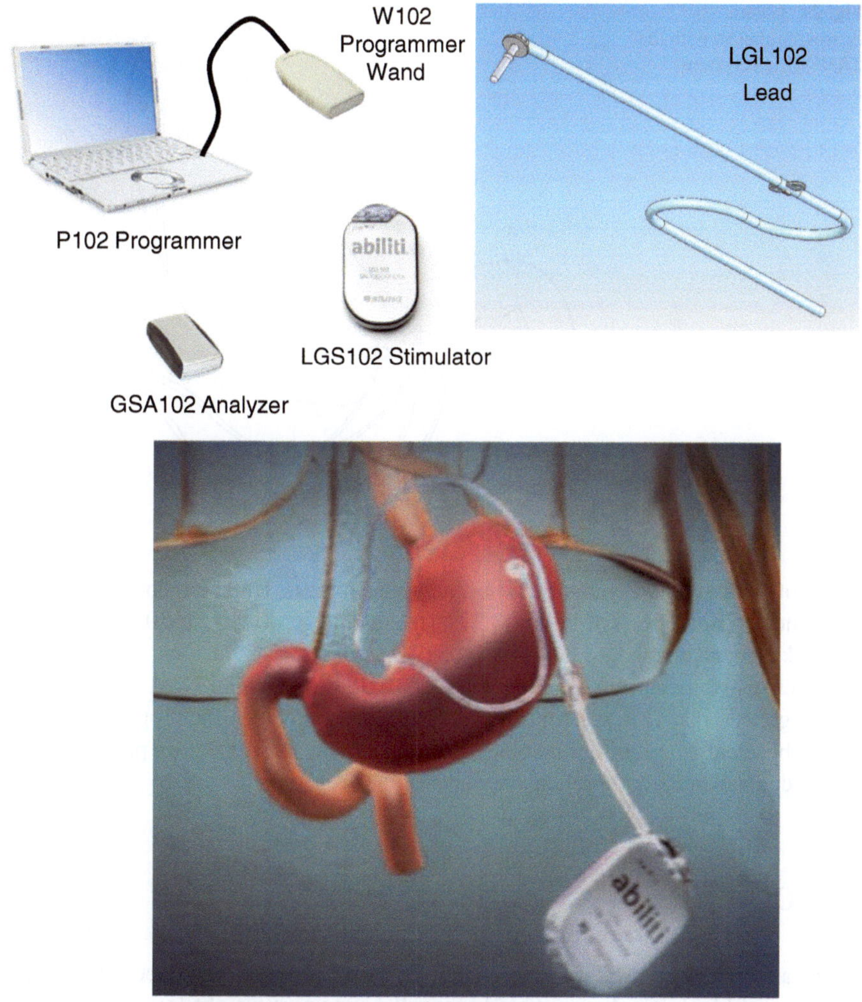

Fig. 23 Gastric neurostimulation with the ABILITI System

term efficacy and safety data. Methods: Data from 57 T2DM patients (30F, BMI 37±4 kg/m^2), inadequately controlled by oral anti-diabetic medications, who were implanted with the TANTALUS for 2 years or more, were analyzed. The risk profile associated with the procedure and the treatment was generated from adverse event (AE) reports; while the metabolic benefit included effects on parameters such as HbA1c, weight, blood pressure and lipids. Results: Procedure related AE such as pain, discomfort, and pocket inflammation were anticipated and considered a part of the healing process. All procedure related AE were resolved within the post-operative period. Device related events, mainly sensation during stimulation, were resolved by simple device reprogramming. None of the subjects was explanted due to adverse events or system malfunction. Six months data demonstrate clinically significant improvement in all metabolic parameters. This effect was maintained in

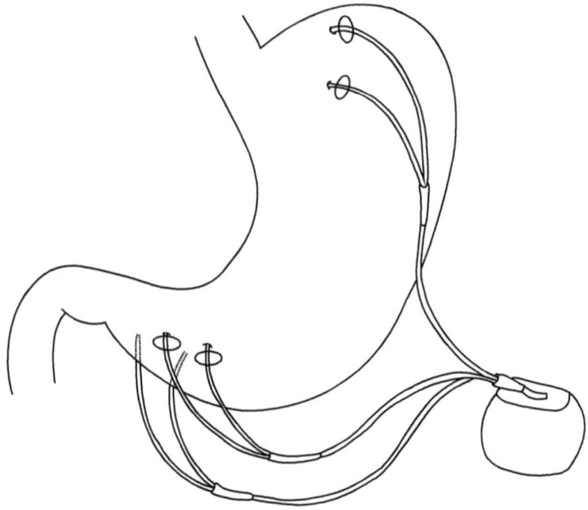

Fig. 24 Gastric neurostimulation with the TANTALUS System

89 % of the patients 2 years post implantation (n=29). HbA1c or body weight or both showed reductions of up to –3.3 % (mean change –0.9 %, P<0.05) and of up to -16 kg (mean change –4.8 kg, P<0.05) respectively. Conclusions: The long term comprehensive metabolic benefits of TANTALUS therapy for T2DM obese patients outweigh its risks. This system offers a viable alternative treatment option for moderate obese patients failing on conservative treatment for T2DM, by providing glycemic control and a comprehensive metabolic effect.

VBLOC Therapy

Herrera et al. (2011): An active implantable device designed to induce sub-diaphramatic vagal block has demonstrated clinically important weight loss and glycemic control in obese type 2 diabetic (DM2) subjects. Objective: Evaluate weight loss, glycemic control and blood pressure (BP) in obese subjects with DM2 or with both DM2 and hypertension (HTN) during 12 months of vagal blocking (VBLOC Therapy)®. Methods: Twenty-eight subjects were implanted with the Maestro Rechargeable System at experienced centers. Weight loss, HbA1c and BP were evaluated at 4 and 12 weeks and 6 and 12 months post-device activation. Results: Baseline demographics were 17 females, 11 males, age 51±2 years and BMI 37±1 kg/m^2 (mean±SE). Twenty five completed 12-months of follow-up. At 4 and 12 weeks and 6 and 12 months, respectively, mean % EWL was 14±2, 21±3, 24±4 and 25±4 % (p<.001); HbA1c decreased by 0.7±0.1, 0.9±0.2, 0.9±0.2 and 1.0±0.2 % from a baseline of 7.8±0.2 % (p<.001); and in DM2 subjects with elevated BP (BP ^{3}130/80 mmHg, n=15), mean arterial pressure decreased by 9±3 (p=.02), 9±2 (p<.001), 13±2 (p<.001) and 8±3 mmHg (p=.03) from a baseline of 98±3 mmHg.

Conclusions: In obese DM2 subjects, VBLOC Therapy was associated with significant weight loss, improvements in HbA1c and reductions in BP in hypertensive subjects. Parameter Week 4 week 12 Month 6 month 12; EWL % (n=25) 14±2 21±3 24±4 25±4; HbA1c % (n=25) 7.1±.1 6.8±.1 6.8±.1 6.6±.1; MAP (mmHg, n=15) 91±3.

NOTES Bariatric Surgery

Principles

NOTES surgery has many potential indications in bariatric procedures. The most current application is the NOTES sleeve gastrectomy using the transvaginal approach, in order to reduce the number of trocars. Single access surgery is competing with it, as well as micro-instrumentation, and it is difficult to predict which approach will prevail. For instance, the experience of a French team shows that most

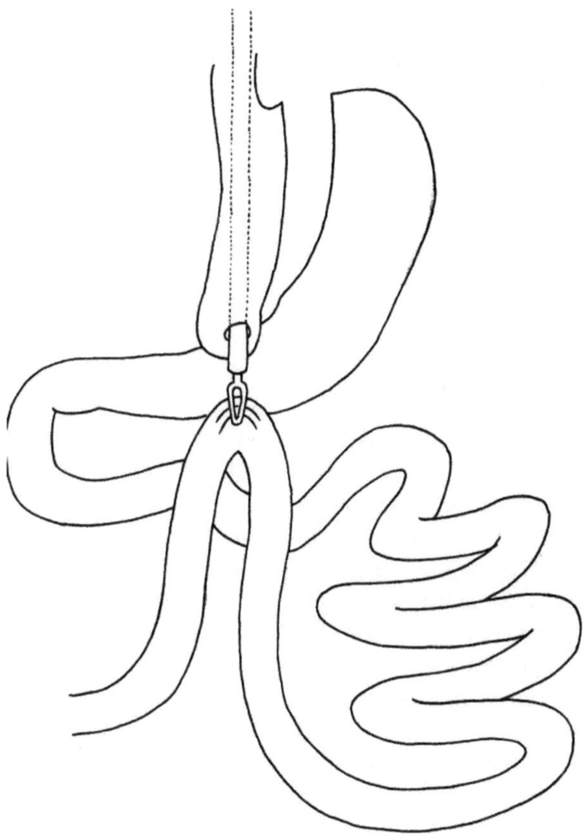

Fig. 25 Totally intragastric NOTES as it could be imagined for a bypass procedure

surgeons can hesitate over the choice of a routine procedure, evolve over the time, and sometimes use mixed approaches Vix et al. (2011).

One may conceive an evolution towards a“true” NOTES procedure, and it would entail a totally intragastric approach for instance. Instruments making it possible to perform an intra-gastric gastro-jejunostomy are being tested, but none has come out for the time being. Endoscopic high-end tools such as the Anubis from Karl Storz (see section “Anubis”) could be the spearhead of this kind of operation.

NOTES Sleeve Gastrectomy

Principles

The laparoscopic SG is established as a one-step procedure in morbid patients. The natural orifice transluminal endoscopic surgical (NOTES) procedures are also gaining in popularity. The transvaginal insertion of instruments (or optical devices) allows a less invasive approach that is competing with single incision approaches. First experiences with hybrid NOTES transvaginal cholecystectomies have been transferred to SG.

Similarities

The transvaginal access is a questionable approach, which has gained popularity in many countries, competing and/or being combined with the SILS approach.

Results

Utech et al. (2011): Describe a small series of SGs for morbid obesity using the vagina as the natural orifice in the form of a hybrid NOTES transvaginal SG. Method: After informing the patient about the experimental nature of this novel technique and our previous experience with laparoscopic transvaginal cholecystectomy, the hybrid NOTES transvaginal SG was performed according to Ramos et al. (2008). Results: Between January 2009 and December 2010 hybrid NOTES transvaginal SG was performed in 16 female patients with an obesity grade II-III. The average age was 42 years (32–50) and the mean BMI 39.3 kg/m^2 (35.5–46.8). The transvaginal technique allowed the reduction of the required ports to an average number of 3.2. The mean operation time was 98 min (75–140). The intraoperative preparation regarding transvaginal assistance was limited due to the intra-abdominal fat distribution. In all cases the specimen was extracted via the transvaginal access. In one case an ovarian teratoma was observed. Postoperatively no pain, bleeding or infection occurred in the part of the transvaginal access. A major complication - proximal leakage - occurred in one patient. There was no mortality. Conclusion: These data demonstrate that the method is feasible but still faces issues. Preparation of the stomach or creating the stapler line was not possible transvaginally in all patients. One reason was the pronounced intra-abdominal fat distribution, which did not allow exposing the upper abdomen without continuously changing the patients between Trendelenburg and anti-Trendelenburg position. For a final establishment of a hybrid NOTES transvaginal SG, longer transvaginal ports and longer staplers have to be developed.

References

Bohdjalian A, Tantalus Research Group (2011) Favorable risk-benefit profile for the TANTALUS® Systel, a meal-initiated therapy to treat T2DM, Medical University of Vienna, Surgery, Vienna (abstract IFSO Hamburg, Sept 2011)

Herrera MF, Toouli J, Kulseng B et al (2011) Treatment of obesity related comorbidities with VBLOC therapy. Instituto Nacional de la Nutricion Salvador Zubrian (INNSZ), Mexico City, Australian Institute of Weight Control, Bedford Park, Australia, St. Olavs Hospital, Trondheim, Australian Institute of Weight Control, Baulkham Hills, University Hospital Basel, Basel, EnteroMedics Inc., St. Paul, University of Minnesota, Minneapolis (abstract IFSO Hamburg, September 2011)

Ramos AC, Zundel N, Neto MG et al (2008) Human hybrid NOTES transvaginal sleeve gastrectomy: initial experience. Surg Obes Relat Dis 4:660–663

Seyfried F, Horbach T, Meyer G et al (2011) Effective modification of eating behaviour and weight-loss using ABILITI® System in obese subjects. University Hospital Wuerzburg, Department of General and Visceral Surgery, Wuerzburg, Imperial College London, Hammersmith Hospital, Dpt. of Investigative Medicine, London, Adipositaszentrum Erlangen-Schwabach, Stadtkrankenhaus Schwabach, Allgemein-, Viszeralchirurgie, Schwabach, Wolfart Klinik München, Zentrum für Adipositas und Metabolische Chirurgie, Munich (abstract IFSO Hamburg, Sept 2011)

Shikora SA (2011) Current state of neuromodulation in the treatment of obesity and other metabolic disorders. Tufts Medical Center, Surgery, Boston (abstract IFSO Hamburg, Sept 2011)

Utech M, Halter J, Knapp A et al (2011) Hybrid NOTES transvaginal sleeve gastrectomy: initial experience of a small consecutive series. Klinikum Vest; Knappschaftskrankenhaus Recklinghausen, Klinik für Allgemein- und Viszeralchirurgie, Recklinghausen (abstract IFSO Hamburg, Sept 2011)

Vix M, Constantino F, Wall J et al (2011) Minimizing abdominal access ports in sleeve gastrectomy: evolution of techniques using NOTES, single port and single incision. IRCAD, Strasbourg (abstract IFSO 2011, Hamburg)

O

Overstitch Endoscopic Suturing System (OESS)

Principles

The Overstitch Endoscopic Suturing System or OESS (Apollo Endosurgery®) is a device which is placed on the gastroscope and permits the suturing by endoluminal approach.

Similarities

This device permits the endoluminal sutures like others, that are used as re-do procedures (see sections "Restore Suturing System (TRIM Procedure)," "Spiderman," and "Flexible Endostitch").

Results

C Thompson presented at 1st Non Inva Congress (Lyon 2011) the first series of 22 patients treated. The patients were previously submitted to RYGB and presented a dilatation of the gastric pouch and/or gastrojejunostomy. Eleven patients underwent to gastrojejunostomy reduction using the OESS, and the post-stomal diameter obtained was 5.6 ± 1.9 mm (78 % reduction), with a median number of three stitches (1–7) placed. Eleven other patients underwent a gastric pouch reduction with placement of a median number of two stitches (range 1–5). At mean follow-up of 3 months, a 60.3 % of weight regain reduction was obtained and % EWL was 21.5 %.

J. Dargent, *Innovative Technologies and Non-Invasive Procedures in Bariatric Surgery*,
DOI 10.1007/978-2-8178-0404-0_12, © Springer-Verlag France 2013

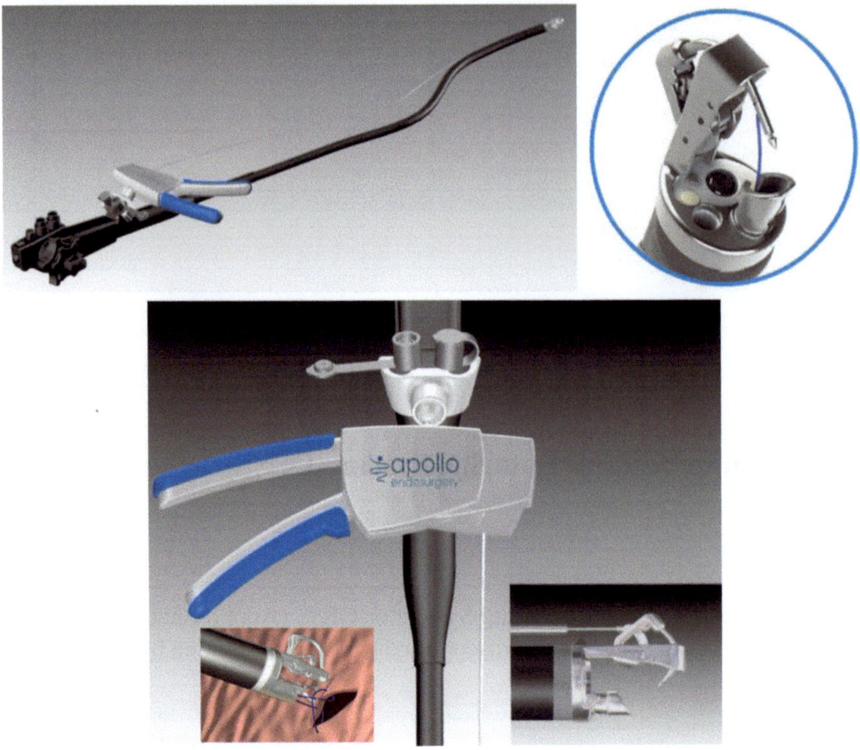

Fig. 26 Apollo System

OVESCO System

(see section "Endoscopic Re-do for Failed Gastric Bypass")

PQ

PEG Drainage

Percutaneous Endoscopic Gastrostomy is commonly used in several indications (e.g. cancerology) for feeding patients unable to swallow. It has potential applications in bariatric surgery in a drainage function, that are tested at the moment. It is yet too early to report on current trials.

POSE Technique

(see section “Transport G-Prox “ROSE” for Re-do After Failed Fastric Bypass and “POSE” for Primary Cases”)

Powered Stapling Device

Principles

Such devices aim at simplifying endoscopic stapling as performed in gastric bypass or sleeve gastrectomy, and/or maximizing security.

Example

The Powered Ethicon Endo-Surgery Echelon FlexTM Endopath® Stapler is a Powered endocutter with enhanced system-wide compression. Like all Echelon FlexTM Endopath® devices, the Powered Echelon FlexTM Endopath® Stapler delivers

J. Dargent, *Innovative Technologies and Non-Invasive Procedures in Bariatric Surgery*,
DOI 10.1007/978-2-8178-0404-0_13,

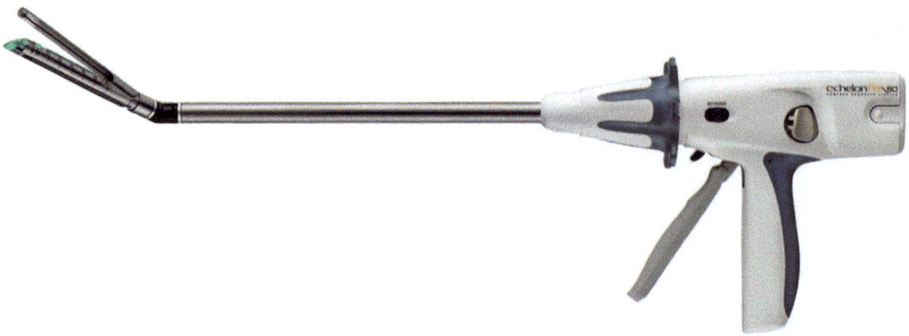

Fig. 27 Powered stapling device (Ethicon)

consistent, properly formed staples for hemostasis across the entire staple line by maintaining a uniform gap in the jaws from the proximal end to the distal tip.

The key-benefit consists in enhanced stability on/near vital structures: this stapler provides virtually effortless firing, allowing the surgeon to reduce inadvertent movement at the end effector by at least 63 % during transection of thick tissue. The firing can be paused or reversed at any time during the transection. The manual closure allows precise placement and tactile feedback as the device is closed. The stapler also offers a dual safety system including both a knife reverse and a manual override. Another manufacturer dedicated to stapling instruments, COVIDIEN, has developed a similar device.

Pressure Guided Adjustments After Laparoscopic Adjustable Band

Principles

A great variability of long-term results of adjustable gastric bands is reported throughout the world. There are several reasons for such differences, such as regional/ethnic differences, expectations set up among individual patients as well as among a larger population groups. A great variability is reported as well in adjustment strategies ending in objectively unmeasurable, uncomparable degrees of restriction achieved during the entire p eriod of bariatric treatment. Pressure guided adjustments which have been proven to deliver similarly accurate information as manometries could be capable of providing more physiological adjustments. This feature may help to enhance the effectiveness and safety of gastric bands mainly due to fine tuning adjustments in more objective way as well as being able to detect even at that time clinically silent, early stages of band, esophageal and gastric disorders which, if not treated adequately usually end-up in complications necessitating reoperation. Pressure guided, physiological adjustments mean that the band should preserve the patient anatomy and the physiological status of esophagus and stomach. Therefore pressure applied by the

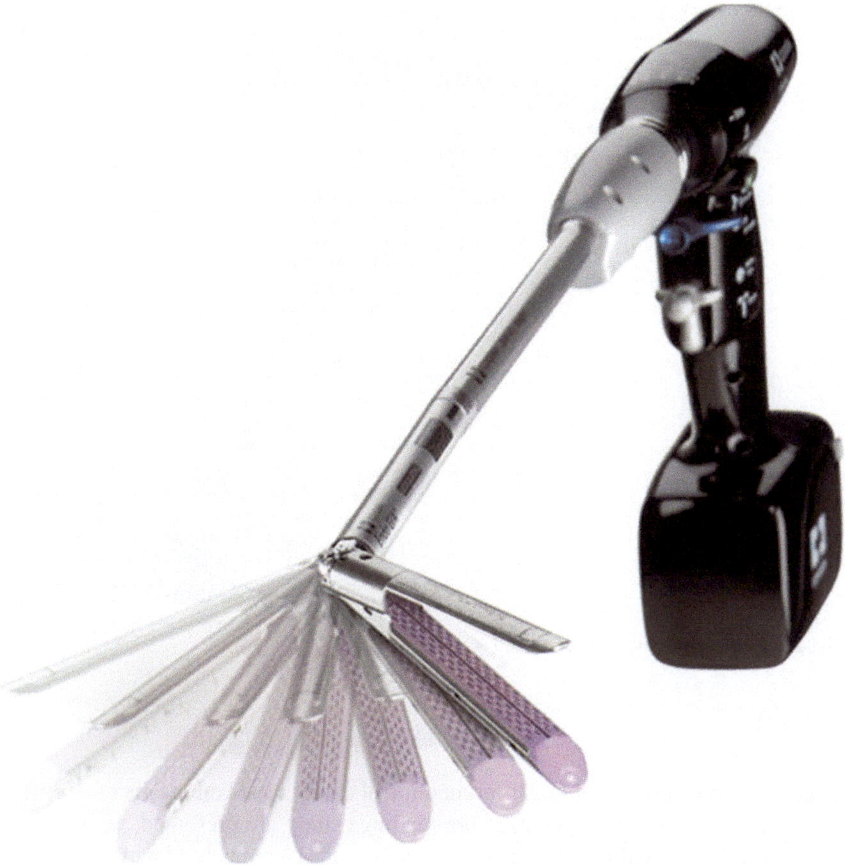

Fig. 28 Powered stapling device (Covidien)

band at stoma region does not adversely affect normal peristaltic activity (propulsive capability) of abdominal esophagus and stomach pouch. Through the means of pressure readings early signs of esophageal or stomach pouch dilatation may be detected with a very similar accuracy compared to e.g. esophageal manometry. Technical failures of the band system can be easily detected as well.

Similarities

Pressure adjustment is supposed not only to match, but to take over fluoroscopy, that is the standard way to perform band adjustments nowadays. The access to the radiology department is an issue in most centers, and this device would prove far more accurate than "in the office adjustments". Yet the problem is to get a sufficient precision, in order to differentiate for instance pouch and esophageal dilatation.

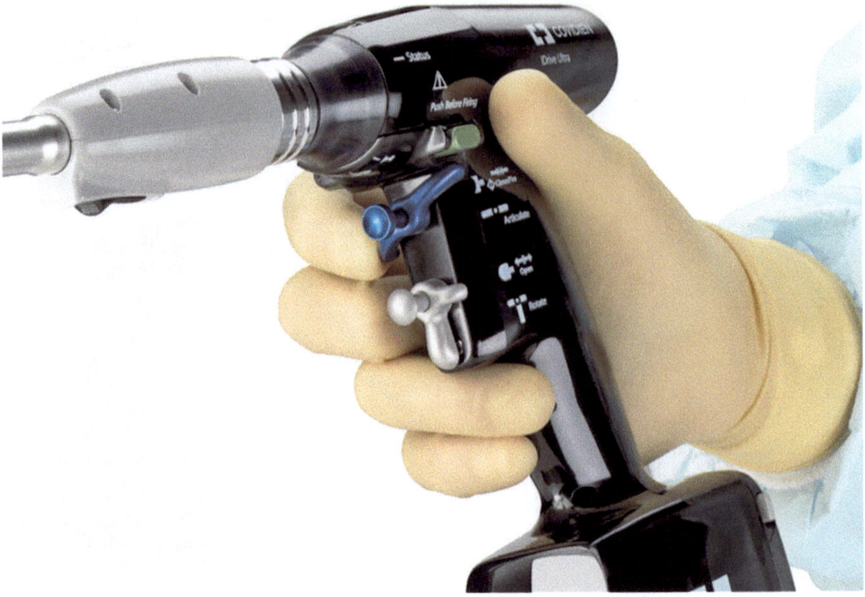

Fig. 29 Powered stapling device, detail (Covidien)

Results

Fried and Dolezalova (2011): Different clinical cases, based on results of a prospective, randomized multi-centre pressure readings study are presented, with focus on common gastric banding complications, such as gastric pouch dilatation/band slippage as well as on over- and under-restriction providing a view on how swift detection and correction is enabled through pressure adjustment readings. Pressure guided adjustments and measurements make it possible to detect precisely and early certain band-related pathologies/irregularities such as band overfilling (over-restriction), band-tubing disconnection (kinking), esophageal motility dysfunctions, esophageal dilatation, pouch dilatation, band slippage and others. Thus in gastric banding patients it may be possible to achieve more physiology in adjustments, resulting in early pathology detection, less complications, and potentially higher overall weight-loss.

Reference

Fried M, Dolezalova K (2011) Pressure guided adjustments after laparoscopic adjustable gastric band. OB Klinika & 1st Faculty of Medicine, Charles University, Centre for Treatment of Obesity and Metabolic Disorders, Prague (abstract IFSO Hamburg, Sept 2011)

R

Reshape Intra Gastric Balloon

(see section "Double Intra Gastric Balloon")

Restore Suturing System (TRIM Procedure)

Principles

The RESTORe Suturing System (Bard®) is a device which covers the gastroscope and permits the reduction of the gastric volume by performing different sutures. These sutures are passed in full thickness method under gastroscopic view into the gastric wall close to the small curvature, from cardia to incisura angularis. Finally they are tied together and create an endoluminal tunnel.

Similarities

This procedure is similar in final shape to the endoluminal tunnel created by stapling (see section "TOGa Device"). It differs from it because only sutures are passed and tied in the stomach, and no endoluminal staplers are used.

Results

Fogel R et al. (2008) reported the experience of this procedure in 64 patients. The procedure time was 45 min and the mean 12-month Excess Weight Loss was

J. Dargent, *Innovative Technologies and Non-Invasive Procedures in Bariatric Surgery*,
DOI 10.1007/978-2-8178-0404-0_14, © Springer-Verlag France 2013

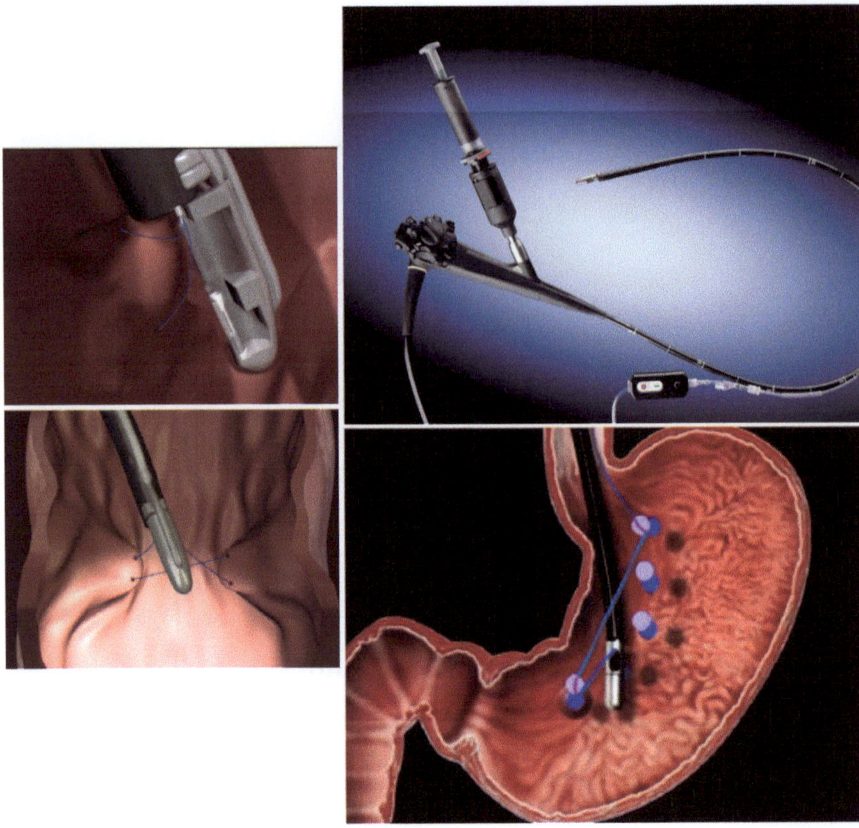

Fig. 30 Restor(e) TRIM procedure

58.1 ± 19.9 %. This procedure was presented by ***C Thompson and S Brethauer at 1st Non Innova Congress (Lyon 2011)*** with the preliminary results of the TRIM trial. In the treatment of 18 patients, they reported a mean procedure time of 125 min and a mean number of six plications (range 4–8) placed per patient. The % EWL achieved in 14 patients after 1 year was 27.7 ± 21.9 %. At 1 year follow-up, a disruption of endoluminal tunnel was found in five patients and partially in eight patients.

Robotic Needle-Holder

Several instruments are on display, for instance the JAIMY®, an instrument matching hand movements, a 5 mm motorized instrument for laparoscopic surgery. It is a hand held motorized articulated instrument designed for the purpose of grasping, retracting, mobilizing, dissecting and suturing of tissues and vessels under endoscopic visualization during surgical procedures. With the handle, surgeon activates three movements simultaneously: total flexion of the shaft, 360° unlimited rotation of the end effector, opening/closing of the jaws. ID-intelligent Dexterity- enables surgeons to extend their hands and to picture movements as if they were inside the patient's body. It is designed to enable surgeons to overcome the unique challenges presented by single incision and conventional laparoscopic surgery. It is reusable, has motorized distal movements for enhanced dexterity and ergonomy. Total flexion is possible for unparalleled access to reach over, under and around structures, as well as unlimited 360° rotation of the end effector at any bending angle for easy suturing and tissue manipulation, with one hand only, intelligent dexterity with seven degrees of freedom (easy triangulation).

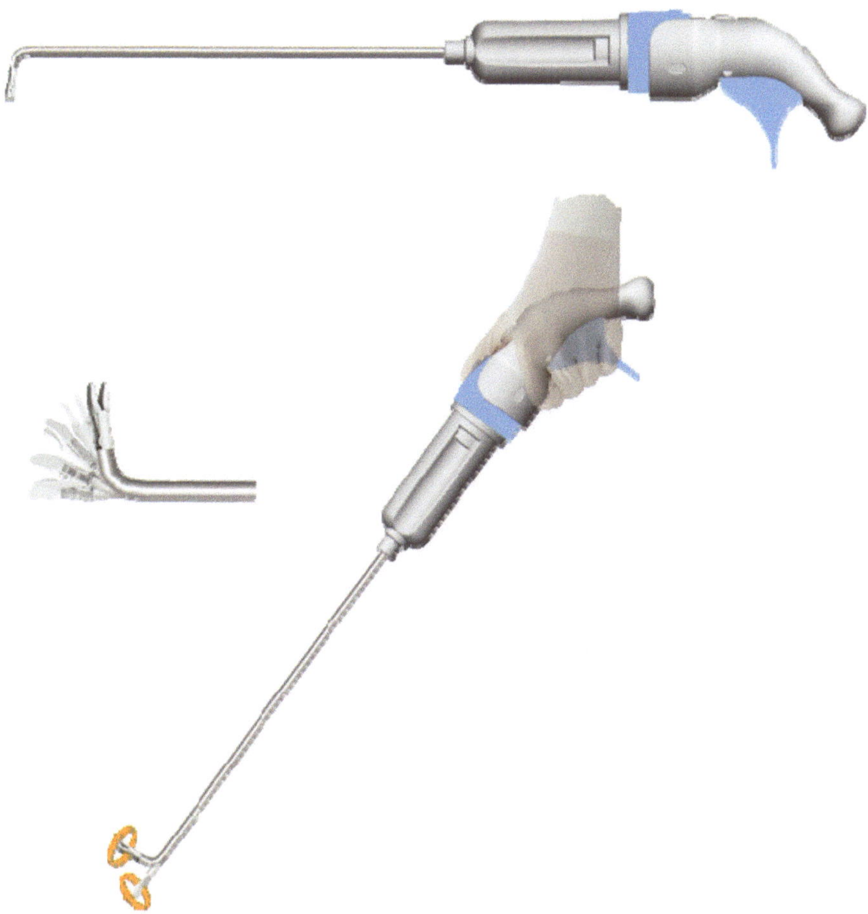

Fig. 31 Jaimy® robotic needle-holder

ROSE Technique

(see section "Transport G-Prox "ROSE" for Re-do After Failed Gastric Bypass and "POSE" for Primary Cases")

Reference

Fogel R, De Fogel J, Bonilla Y et al (2008) Clinical experience of transoral suturing for an endoluminal vertical gastroplasty: 1-year follow-up in 64 patients. Gastrointest Endosc 68:51–58

S

Safestitch Device

This device is inspired by the Stretta procedure (see antireflux procedures: "The use of radiofrequency"), that worked best and created fibrosis and collagen. The Safe Stitch® device realizes a mucosal excision. A suture infolding of excision beds creates a smaller lumen and the deposition of a scar at GE junction and greater curvature. The healing scar tissue increases creep resistance of infold.

SILS Laparoscopic Bilio Pancreatic Diversion

Principles

SILS in bariatric has been showed to be feasible also for other advanced procedures outside of gastric bypass, like Biliopancreatic Diversion, with the same aim of improving the cosmetic outcomes and reducing the abdominal trauma and postoperative pain.

Similarities

The procedure consists in performing the typical biliopancreatic diversion, but maintaining the distal stomach in place. Hence, the access-site remains smaller, because no specimen needs to be removed, and the original umbilical scar can be used.

J. Dargent, *Innovative Technologies and Non-Invasive Procedures in Bariatric Surgery*,
DOI 10.1007/978-2-8178-0404-0_15,

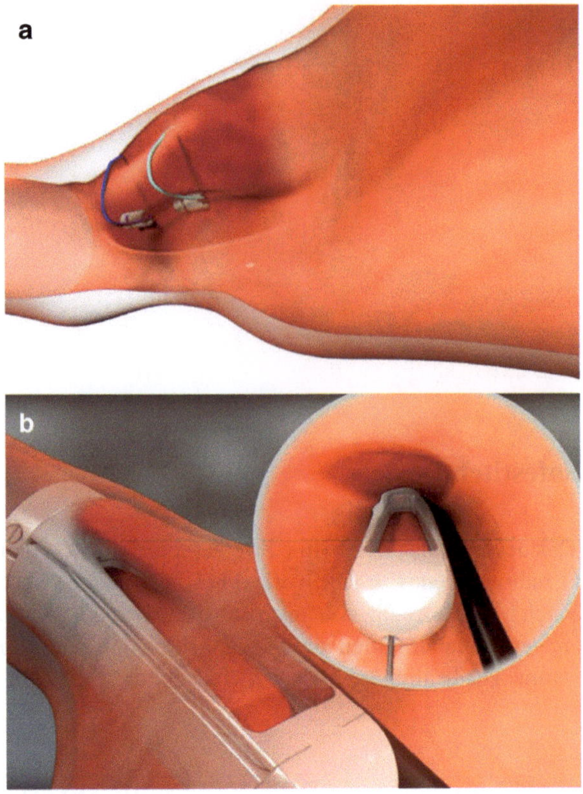

Fig. 32 Safestitch device (**a**) tissue apposition, (**b**) mucosal excision

Results

Tacchino R et al. (2010) reported the first one patient treated through this access, with no conversion to standard laparoscopy and a patient's discharge on 4th postoperative day.

SILS Laparoscopic Gastric Banding

Principles

The procedure consists in the placement of an adjustable gastric banding around the cardia similarly to that performed through classical multi-trocars laparoscopy. The difference is the unique laparoscopic access, which is usually the original umbilical scar. A sub-phrenic access has also been suggested.

Results

Nguyen NT et al. (2008) reported the first patient treated by SILS. Comparative studies between SILS technique and standard five trocars technique have been reported as well. Raman S et al. (2011) showed a significant reduced use of morphine and analgesic drugs in the early postoperative time after SILS. Ayloo SM et al. (2011) found in the group of SILS a pain score value higher at the discharge and reduced at 1 week postoperatively. Saber AA et al. (2010) showed a reduced pain score and analgesia drugs too in the SILS group. Nguyen NT et al. (2010) reported a reduced operative time and blood loss during the SILS technique, besides a 13 % conversion rate to standard laparoscopy. One has demonstrated that the conversion rate was improved by the learning curve, and Galvani C et al. (2012) reported an incidence of 74.2 % in the first 35 patients, 14.2 % in the second 35 patients and 0 % in the last 19 patients treated. Learning curve is fundamental also in reducing the operative time, as shown by Koh et al. (2010).

SILS Laparoscopic Gastric Bypass

Principles

SILS in bariatric has been shown feasible also for advanced procedures which involve the performance of an anastomosis like in gastric bypass. Both one-loop/mini gastric bypass and Roux-en-Y gastric bypass have been reported through SILS. The main purpose remains the improvement of the cosmetic outcomes, besides the reduced postoperative pain and abdominal trauma.

Similarities

The procedure consists in the realization of the same gastric bypass circuit performed with five or more abdominal trocars, but through a single-access, usually at the umbilicus.

Results

Tacchino R et al. (2010) reported the first 14 patients treated by SILS one-loop/mini gastric bypass, with no conversion to standard laparoscopy and an operative time of less than 2 hours.

Huang CK et al. (2009) reported the first patient treated by SILS Roux-en-Y gastric bypass.

Comparative studies between SILS technique and standard five trocars technique have been reported as well. Huang CK et al. (2010) showed a significant higher operative time in the SILS group, but a significant higher scar satisfaction score. Allee JL et al. (2011) presented a significant reduction of pain score at postoperative day 1 and 3, and a reduced C-reactive protein levels at the 4th postoperative day.

SILS Lap-Band Removal

Principles

SILS Lap Band Removal is performed mainly with the reduction of the abdominal trauma in mind, since the patient has already been submitted to laparoscopy and has surgical scars. In order to reduce the abdominal and peritoneal punctures, and probably the risk of future incisional hernias, only one access is used to place the optical system and the instruments into the abdomen.

Similarities

The procedure consists in the removal of the adjustable gastric banding through a unique laparoscopic access, which is the placement of the subcutaneous port, usually located in the left hypocondrium. Thanks to this method, the previous incision at the subcutaneous port is used, but only one abdominal opening is performed in the abdomen.

Results

Dapri G (2012) reported the first ten patients treated through this access, with a laparoscopic time of 26 ± 8.6 min, an operative bleeding of 8 ± 5.5 mL, and no necessity of additional trocar.

SILS Sleeve Gastrectomy

Principles

SILS Sleeve Gastrectomy gained a lot of interest in SILS bariatric because the specimen needs to be removed from the abdomen at the end of the procedure, hence the unique incision in the abdomen can be used to remove the stomach as well. Problems remain, as during the other SILS procedures, the use of the umbilicus as an access in patients with a high BMI (super and super super-obese patients).

Similarities

The procedure consists into performing sleeve gastrectomy in a standard laparoscopical way, but through a single-incision, usually at the umbilicus.

Results

Saber AA et al. (2008) reported the first patient treated by SILS.

Comparative studies between SILS technique and standard five trocars technique have been reported as well. Saber AA et al. (2010) showed a significantly reduced postoperative pain score, and a reduced use of opioid analgesia in the SILS group. Lakdawala MA et al. (2011) found in the SILS group a significantly less important VAS value after the first eight postoperative hours.

SILS Trocars

Single Incision Laparoscopic Surgery (SILS) represents an evolution of classic laparoscopy. Instead of 4–6 trocars inserted in the abdomen through 4–6 skin incisions, only one multiple trocar is used through a single incision, or 3–4 trocars are inserted in the same incision, with a unique access in the abdomen. The main purpose of this evolved approach of laparoscopy is to improve the cosmetic results, because at the end of surgery only one incision appears evident in the abdomen. Randomized studies evaluating postoperative pain, abdominal trauma, hospital stay, patient's satisfaction, early and late postoperative complications have been reported, this procedure being still under investigation.

Spiderman

Principles

The Spiderman (Ethicon, Johnson & Johnson®) is a device designed to be placed on the gastroscope, permitting the endoluminal suturing. It is still under development, but it can be used to reduce the stoma diameter after Roux-en-Y gastric bypass.

Similarities

This device permits the endoluminal sutures like using the RESTORe, the OESS, and the Flexible Endostitch.

Fig. 33 Spiderman System

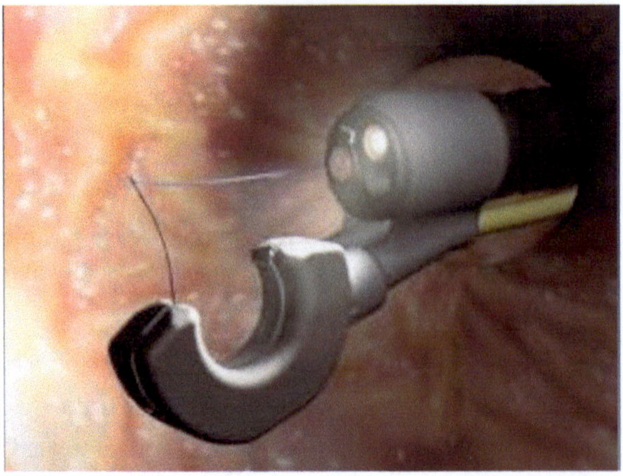

Results

A Torquati showed at ***25thASMBS Congress (Washington DC, 2008***) the benefits of this device, passing 1-3 sutures around the dilated gastrojejunostomy. After having placed the device at the level of the stoma under gastroscopic control, a stitch encircles the stoma and an external knot is pushed down to close the suture, with the final result of reducing the stoma diameter. A Torquati presented at ***1st Non Inva Congress (Lyon 2011)*** the preliminary results in nine patients, with a stoma diameter reduction from 19 ± 2.5 to 14.5 ± 3.2 mm.

Stents for Staple-Line Leaks

(see section "Endoscopic Treatment of Post-op Complications")

Stomaphyx

Principles

StomaphyX is a natural orifice transluminal endoscopic procedure to reduce gastric pouch size following RYGB.

The StomaphyX (Endogastric Solution®) is an endoscopic device which works like an overtube for the gastroscope. It allows the suction of the gastric wall in full thickness method, and the placement of polypropilene fasteners at the base of the tissue that has been suctioned. Basically, StomaphyX improves the restriction compartment, treating a dilated gastric pouch with weight regain in patients who underwent a previous RYGB.

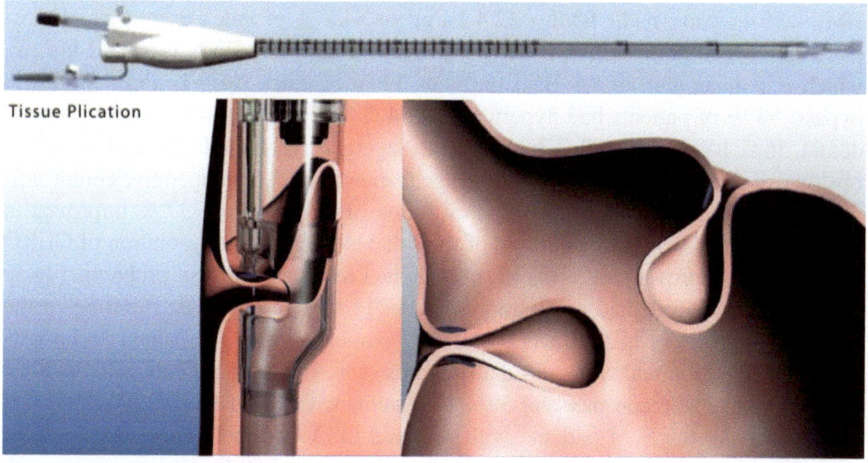

Fig. 34 Stomaphyx System

Similarities

The system is unique in its mechanism and it is not similar to other endoluminal procedures. Yet the purpose is to fight weight-regain after gastric bypass, alongside other procedures herein described (see sections "Restore Suturing System (TRIM Procedure)" and "ROSE Technique").

Results

Mikami DJ et al. (2010) reported the preliminary results in 36 patients with previous RYGB. After 6 months the patients presented a weight loss of 8.7 kg, and after 1 year of 10 kg. Moreover, eight patients suffering of gastro-esophageal reflux diseases before the procedure, had an improvement of their symptoms at follow-up. Similarly, Leitman IM et al. (2010) reported a mean weight loss of 7.3 kg after a mean follow-up of 5.8 months in 64 patients with RYGB. All symptoms from dumping syndrome to gastroesophageal reflux were improved in a similar way. Monouchehri N et al. (2011) reported also the feasibility of the use of StomaphyX in patients with previous vertical banded gastroplasty, reporting a drop of BMI from 43.4±9.7 to 39.8±9.1 kg/m^2. Finally, in literature few cases of fistula closure by StomaphyX have been reported as well (Overcash et al. 2008; Schweitzer et al. 2009).

A comprehensive report has been published recently by S Ahmed and JM Morton (2011): At a single academic institution, between 2008 and 2010, 11 patients underwent StomaphyX. BMI and comorbidities before and after RYGB and StomaphyX procedures, and complications following surgery were recorded. Results: Of 11 patients, 82 % were women. Mean demographics are as follows: age at RYGB – 42.8 years; age at StomaphyX – 47.1 years; 60.7 months between procedures; index

BMI – 56.4 kg/m^2; nadir BMI – 32.4 kg/m^2 or 84.7 % of index excess weight lost (%EWL). Mean preoperative BMI at the time of the StomaphyX was 41.2 kg/ m^2, which is a mean gain of 8.8 BMI units, or 32 % of index %EWL. Prior to gastric bypass, 54 % of patients had hypertension, 54 % had diabetes, 45 % had hyperlipidemia, 36 % had GERD, 82 % had musculoskeletal (msk) complaints, and 64 % had obstructive sleep apnoea (OSA); on average, patients had 3.5 preoperative comorbidities. At 1 year, 66 % of patients had resolution of hypertension (37 % improved in hypertension), 100 % had resolution of their diabetes, 50 % had resolution of GERD (the rest had improvement of GERD), 22 % had resolution of msk problems (44 % improved), and 86 % had resolution of OSA (14 % improved). At the time of the StomaphyX, patients had an average of 2.27 comorbidities. One patient had a new onset of diabetes; no other case of diabetes was seen. 100 % of patients with resolved msk problems had recurrence and 50 % of patients with improved msk problems had worsened pain. 67 % of patients with resolved OSA had recurrence. 50 % of the patients with recurrent msk problems had resolution, and 50 % of the patients with worsened msk problems improved. 100 % of patients with recurrent OSA had resolution. Compared to an average LOS of 3.1 days following gastric bypass, patients were discharged on the same day as their StomaphyX procedure. Of the 11 patients, only one patient suffered a complication (perforated ulcer). By 2 weeks post StomaphyX, patients lost an average of 12 % of their pre-StomaphyX EWL (n=9).

Conclusion: As early as 2 weeks, patients undergoing StomaphyX lose 12 % of their excess weight. The minimally invasive nature of StomaphyX, elimination of overnight hospitalization and low complication rates makes it a safe alternative for treating insufficient weight loss and recurrence of comorbidities post RYGB.

References

Ahmed S, Morton JM (2011) Does STOMAPHYX treat weight gain and comorbidity recurrence following RYGB? Stanford University, Surgery, Stanford, USA. Abstract IFSO Hamburg, Sept 2011

Ayloo SM, Buchs NC, Addeo P et al (2011) Traditional versus single-site placement of adjustable gastric banding: a comparative study and cost analysis. Obes Surg 21:815–819

Dapri G (2012) Specially designed curved reusable instruments for single-access laparoscopy: 2.5-year experience in 265 patients. Minim Invasive Ther Allied Technol 21:31–39

Demyttenaere SV, Bergman S, Pham T et al (2010) Transoral incisionless fundoplication for gastroesophageal reflux disease in an unselected patient population. Surg Endosc 24:854–858

Galvani CA, Gallo AS, Gorodner MV (2012) Single-incision and dual-incision laparoscopic adjustable gastric band: evaluation of initial experience. Surg Obes Relat Dis 8:194–200

Huang CK, Houng JY, Chiang CJ et al (2009) Single incision transumbilical laparoscopic Roux-en-Y gastric bypass: a first case report. Obes Surg 19:1711–1715

Huang CK, Lo CH, Houng JY et al (2012) Surgical results of single-incision transumbilical laparoscopic Roux-en-Y gastric bypass. Surg Obes Relat Dis 8:201–207

Koh CE, Martin DJ, Cavallucci DJ et al (2011) On the road to single-site laparoscopic adjustable gastric banding: lessons learned from 60 cases. Surg Endosc 25:947–953

Lakdawala MA, Muda NH, Goel S et al (2011) Single-incision sleeve gastrectomy versus conventional laparoscopic sleeve gastrectomy--a randomised pilot study. Obes Surg 21:1664–1670

Leitman IM, Virk CS, Avgerinos DV et al (2010) Early results of trans-oral endoscopic plication and revision of the gastric pouch and stoma following Roux-en-Y gastric bypass surgery. JSLS 14:217–220

Manouchehri N, Birch DW, Menzes C et al (2011) Natural orifice surgery: endoluminal pouch reduction following failed vertical banded gastroplasty. Obes Surg 21:1787–1791

Nguyen NT, Hinojosa MW, Smith BR et al (2008) Single laparoscopic incision transabdominal (SLIT) surgery-adjustable gastric banding: a novel minimally invasive surgical approach. Obes Surg 18:1628–1631

Nguyen NT, Slone J, Reavis K (2010) Comparison study of conventional laparoscopic gastric banding versus laparoendoscopic single site gastric banding. Surg Obes Relat Dis 6:503–507

Overcash WT (2008) Natural orifice surgery (NOS) using StomaphyX for repair of gastric leaks after bariatric revisions. Obes Surg 18:882–885

Raman SR, Franco D, Holover S et al (2011) Does transumbilical single incision laparoscopic adjustable gastric banding result in decreased pain medicine use? A case-matched study. Surg Obes Relat Dis 7:129–133

Saber AA, Elgamal MH, Itawi EA et al (2008) Single incision laparoscopic sleeve gastrectomy (SILS): a novel technique. Obes Surg 18:1338–1342

Saber AA, El-Ghazaly TH, Elain A et al (2010) Single-incision laparoscopic placement of an adjustable gastric band versus conventional multiport laparoscopic gastric banding: a comparative study. Am Surg 76:1328–1332

Saber AA, El-Ghazaly TH, Dewoolkar AV et al (2010) Single-incision laparoscopic sleeve gastrectomy versus conventional multiport laparoscopic sleeve gastrectomy: technical considerations and strategic modifications. Surg Obes Relat Dis 6:658–664

Schweitzer M, Steele K, Mitchell M et al (2009) Transoral endoscopic closure of gastric fistula. Surg Obes Relat Dis 5:283–284

Tacchino RM, Greco F, Matera D (2010) Single-incision laparoscopic biliopancreatic diversion. Surg Obes Relat Dis 6:444–445

Tacchino RM, Greco F, Matera D et al (2010) Single-incision laparoscopic gastric bypass for morbid obesity. Obes Surg 20:1154–1160

TU

TANTALUS Device

(See section "Neuromodulation in Obesity Treatments")

TERIS Device

Principles

The Transoral Endoscopic Restrictive Implant System (TERIS) is a new endoscopic procedure: the gastric wall is plicated, and full thickness perforated and silicon anchors are passed. Five silicon anchors are placed on the whole circumference of the fundus, and finally a central restrictor is attached to the stapled plications across the anchors. The system was developed through the collaboration between Barosense® and the University of Laval in Quebec (Canada), and after the first prototype, the second generation was developed.

Similarities

This procedure is unique in its technique and it represents a restrictive procedure similar to an internal gastric band. Inserting a device at the GE junction has also been attempted with other materials (see section "Full Sense System for Obesity"), and could compete with the injection of biocompatible material (see section "HA Injection at the GE Junction").

J. Dargent, *Innovative Technologies and Non-Invasive Procedures in Bariatric Surgery*,
DOI 10.1007/978-2-8178-0404-0_16, © Springer-Verlag France 2013

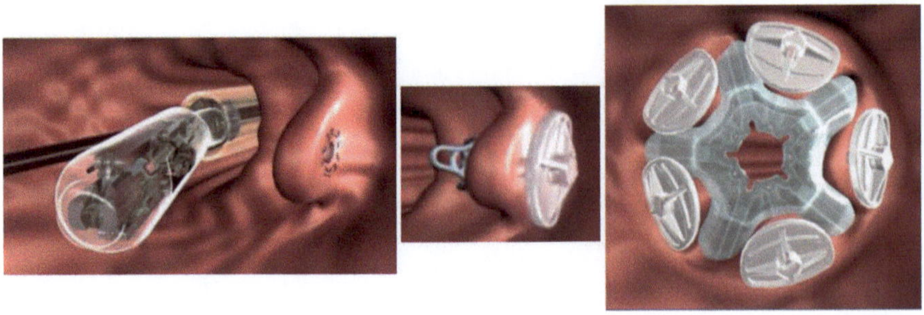

Fig. 35 TERIS System

Results

Biertho L et al. (2010) reported the preliminary results in 12 patients. The BMI dropped from 43.7 kg/m^2 (range 38–48) to 30.6±4.7 after 12 months, and the % EWL at 9 months was 45 %. Due to the appearance of restrictor device blockage, the system evolved and ***S Biron at 1st Non Inva Congress (Lyon 2011)*** presented the results of the second group of ten patients treated, with a % EWL of 38 % at 18 months.

TOGa Device

Principles

The TOGa (Satiety®) is a TransOral Gastroplasy and it consists in a set of transoral endoscopically guided staplers used to create a stapled restrictive pouch along the lesser curve of the stomach. The TOGa sleeve stapler is like an overtube, the gastroscope being accommodated inside and pushed in the upper part of the stomach. Once in the stomach, the stapler jaws are opened and the tissue is acquired in the device thanks to the suction copmpartment of the device, and staplers are fired (two rows usually). A 8–9 cm long endoluminal tunnel with a 19 mm diameter is finally created.

Similarities

This sleeve stapler creates a restrictive procedure similar to the vertical banded gastroplasty (VBG) performed in open surgery, with the difference that it is completely endoscopic and that no band (or other restrictive device) is placed at the outlet.

Results

Devière J et al. (2008) reported the feasibility of the TOGa in 21 patients, with a % EWL rate of 24.4 % at 6 months. During the phase II of the pilot trial, a 52 % of

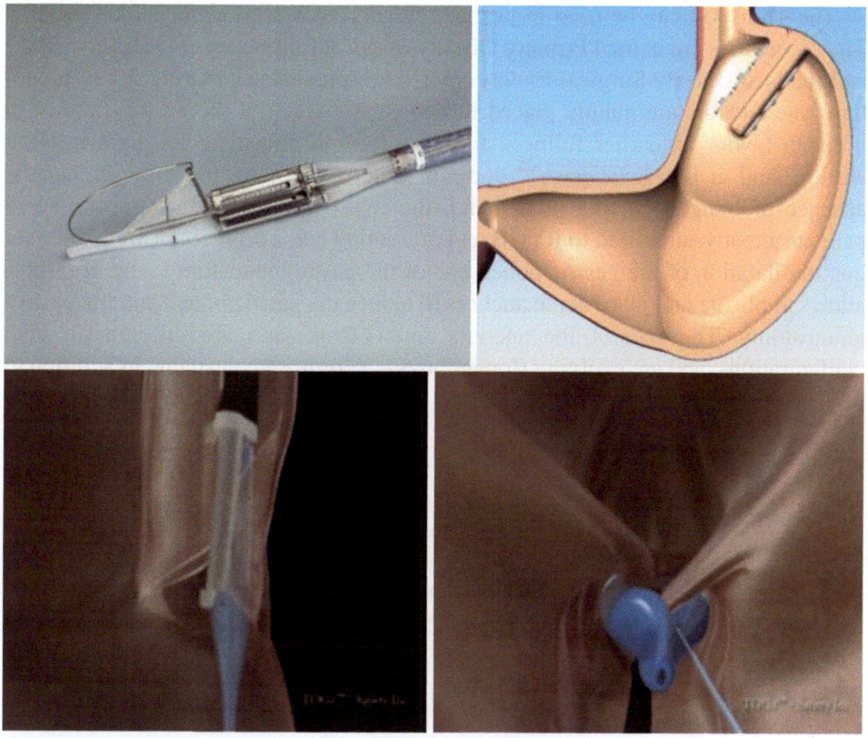

Fig. 36 TOGa System

% EWL was achieved after 24 months in 6 patients. In the European Multicenter Trial, enrolling 87 patients, at 1 year a 41.3 % of % EWL in patients with a BMI>40 kg/m^2 was achieved, and a 52.2 % of % EWL in patients with a BMI<39.9 kg/m^2.

Unfortunately, the company has closed down in 2011 and intended to sell its assets. Although CE mark was available, the company decided not to commercialize the device, while FDA submission (PMA) was pending.

Transport G-Prox "ROSE" for Re-do After Failed Gastric Bypass and "POSE" for Primary Cases

Principles

The Transport (USGI®) is a flexible 4-lm device designed for passing the g-Prox (endoscopic grasper) and the g-Lix (corkscrew-shaped tissue grasper) in the gastric wall in order to place the g-Cath (expandable tissue anchors). This multilumen device works under gastroscopic view, hence the gastroscope is accomodated inside one of the four channels. Once the stomach is plicated in fullthickness by the g-Prox grasper, the anchor (g-Cath) is passed and placed into the tissue using the g-Lix grasper.

The Transport can be used in primary surgery as well as in revisional surgery. The procedures are named Primary Obesity Surgical Endoscopy (POSE procedure) and Revised Obesity Surgical Endoscopy (ROSE procedure). During POSE procedure, the anchors are mainly placed in two gastric areas: at the gastric fundus, in order to favour an earlier fullness and a more rapid transit of the food into the antrum, and at the distal gastric body, in order to prolong the fullness and the absence of hunger. On the other hand, the ROSE procedures are performed in patients already submitted to RYGB and presenting e.g. a problem of weight regain due to dilatation of the gastric pouch and/or the gastrojejunostomy. The Transport allows to plicate and place some anchors to reduce the gastric pouch and the gastrojejunostomy. The size of the anchors and G-Prox jaws are different in both configurations, and are evolving (longer jaws – 33 mm – are available in addition to the 16 mm jaws).

Similarities

The anchors placed at the base of each plication increase the restrictive compartment in a similar way as the fasteners placed during the StomaphyX procedure (see

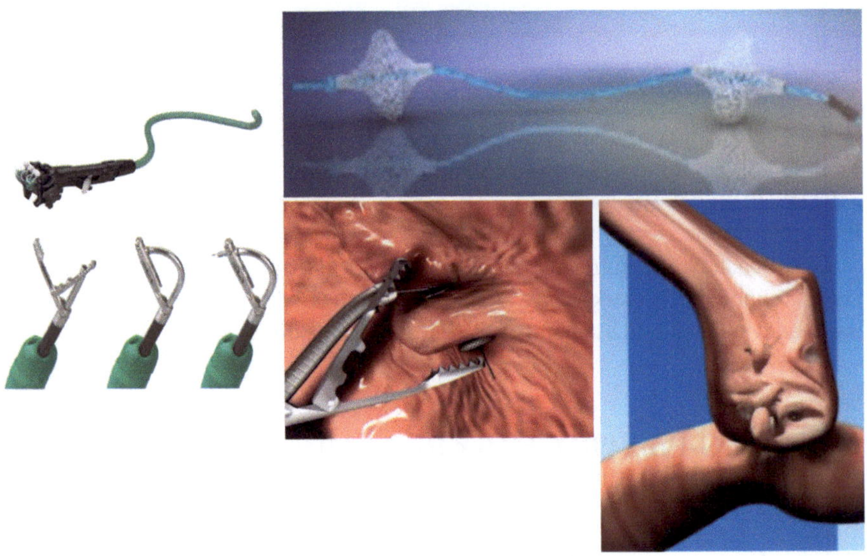

Fig. 37 Transport System

section "Stomaphyx"). The great interest of this device is the access to primary obese patients (in the POSE model), which makes it a strong competitor to any laparoscopic procedure provided its effects can be proved longstanding. Yet a regular and sustained weight-loss at 1 year post-operatively is mandatory in order to achieve such a goal.

Results

G Lopez-Nava presented at 1st Non Inva Congress (Lyon 2011) the results of POSE procedure in 20 patients treated, with an achieved mean weight loss of 10.8 kg and a mean % EWL of 37 %.

T Lavin presented at the XVI IFSO Congress (Hamburg 2011) the results of POSE procedure in 54 patients treated. The mean procedure time was 75 min and the mean number of anchors placed at the fundus was 9.4–13.7, and 3.0 at the distal body. A mean 36.5 ± 35.6 % of % EWL was achieved after 18 months in ten patients, with a 80 % reduced hunger and 60 % earlier satiety.

The results of the ROSE procedure were reported by Horgan S et al. (2010) in a multicenter IRB-approved registry, enrolling 116 patients in nine different hospitals. The interval time between the RYGB and the ROSE procedure was 2 years, the mean total number of anchors placed per case was 5.9, and the mean procedure time was 87 min. A mean 50 % of gastrojejunostomy reduction and a mean 44 % gastric pouch reduction were obtained, with a mean 18 % of % EWL and a mean 32 % of weight regain lost. Furthermore, the ROSE procedure stopped weight regain in 88 % of the patients. Similarly Raman SR et al. (2011) reported in 37 patients a gastrojejunostomy diameter reduction, from 21.5 to 10 mm, and a 23.5 ± 66.4 % of % EWL after a mean follow-up of 4.6 months.

Transpyloric Shuttle® (Baronova)

The BAROnova® technology consists of a TransPyloric Shuttle device that is inserted into the stomach through the mouth using a simple out-patient endoscopic procedure (10 min). Likewise, removal can be accomplished in 15 min. Once in place, the TransPyloric Shuttle may cause a patient's stomach to fill up faster, stay full longer, and potentially delay gastric emptying, which is a known mechanism of action for weight loss Clarkton et al. (1997).

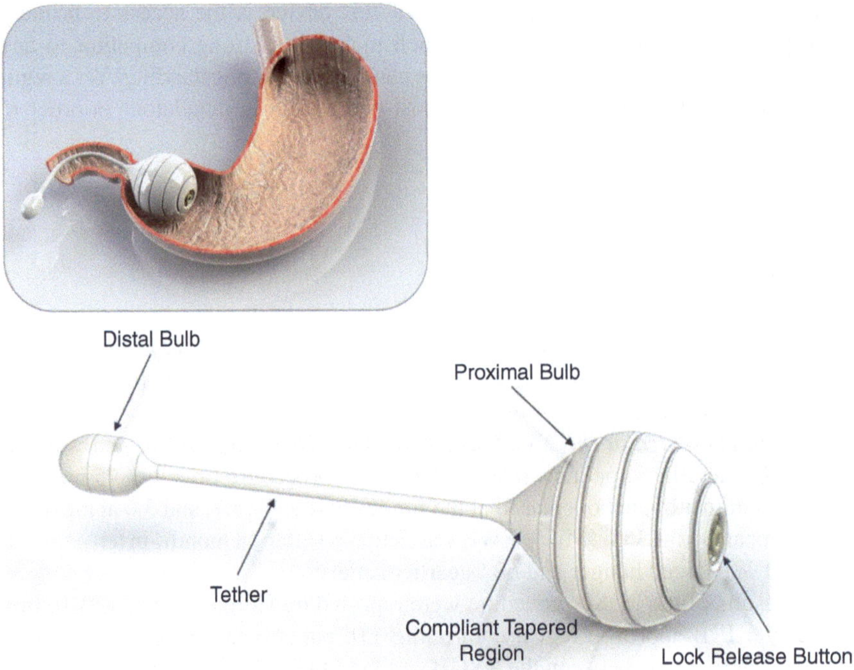

Fig. 38 (**a**, **b**) Excision and healing create tissue apposition

References

Biertho L, Hould FS, Lebel S et al (2010) Transoral endoscopic restrictive implant system: a new endoscopic technique for the treatment of obesity. Surg Obes Relat Dis 6:203–205

Clarkton WK, Pantano MM, Morley JE et al (1997) Evidence for the anorexia of aging; gastroinestinal transit and hunger in healthy elderly vs. young adults. Am J Physiol 272(1 Pt 2): R243–R248

Devière J, Ojeda Valdes G, Cuevas Herrera L et al (2008) Safety, feasibility and weight loss after transoral gastroplasty: First human multicenter study. Surg Endosc 22:589–598

Horgan S, Jacobsen G, Weiss GD et al (2010) Incisionless revision of post-Roux-en-Y bypass stomal and pouch dilation: multicenter registry results. Surg Obes Relat Dis 6:290–295

Raman SR, Holover S, Garber S (2011) Endolumenal revision obesity surgery results in weight loss and closure of gastric-gastric fistula. Surg Obes Relat Dis 7:304–308

VWXYZ

ValenTX System for Morbid Obesity

Principles

The ValenTX® is an endoluminal 80 cm long sleeve-device, which is anchored at the level of the gastroesophageal junction and pushed distally until to reach the first jejunum. The anchors are fixed under endoscopic control, in full thickness method and on the entire circumference of the esophagus. This sleeve-device permits to completely exclude all the stomach and also the first small bowel loops, a restricted quantity of foods to be ingested, and a certain glucose homeostasis barrier in patients suffering of diabetes mellitus.

Similarities

This sleeve-device is unique in its design, but it works similarly to the EndoBarrier Gastrointestinal Liner (GI Dynamics®) in terms of purpose (weight loss/diabetes mellitus improvement) (see section "Duodeno-Jejunal Bypass-Sleeve"). It differs from it because the ValenTX is longer, and it is anchored at the esophagus instead of the first duodenum.

Results

The ValenTX device has been placed in 12 human beings by ***S Horgan and University of California San Diego***. The results were presented at ***2011 SAGES Congress (San Antonio, TX)***. The device was well tolerated with an exception of three patients, who required an early removal, and no significant adverse events

J. Dargent, *Innovative Technologies and Non-Invasive Procedures in Bariatric Surgery*,
DOI 10.1007/978-2-8178-0404-0_17, © Springer-Verlag France 2013

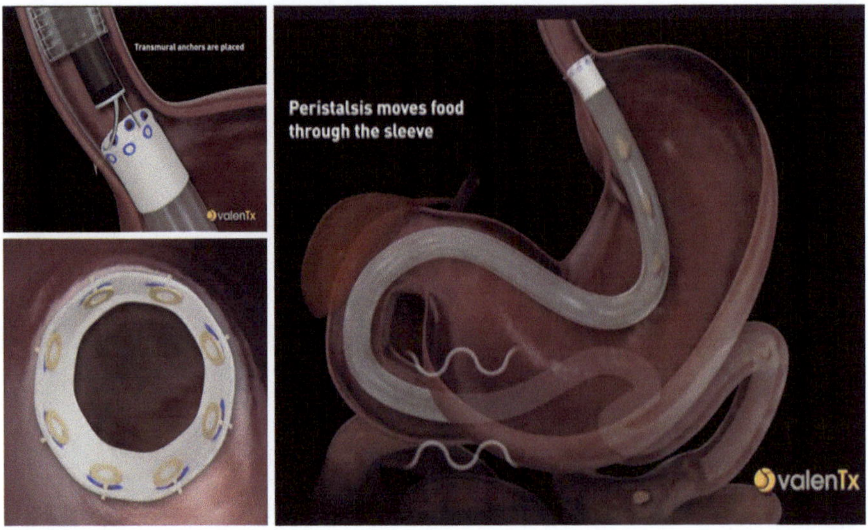

Fig. 39 ValenTX system

were presented; a 40 % of % EWL was registered at 12 weeks after its placement.

VBLOC-Therapy

(See section "Neuromodulation in Obesity Treatments")

Weight Regain due to Dilation of the Gastrojejunostomy After Bypass Surgery

Bariatric surgery is an undisputed option for morbid obesity. However, the long-term failure rate after gastric bypass surgery is 20–35 %, and even higher in super-obese patients (Buchwald et al. 2004). A number of studies suggest that a weight gain may be due to the gradual enlargement of the stomach pouch or due to the dilatation of the gastrojejunal anastomosis because of overeating. Reoperation with reducing the pouch volume or shortening the common loop is one option (Mullady et al. 2009). Given the high morbidity (15 %) and even mortality (1 %) of any surgical intervention in these patients, alternative endoscopic methods have been proposed (Heylen et al. 2010). Many devices presented in this directory have been proved safe and efficacious here (see sections "Overstitch Endoscopic Suturing System," "Spiderman," "Flexible endostitch," and "Restore Suturing System (TRIM Procedure)")

References

Buchwald H, Avidor Y, Braunwald EJ et al (2005) JAMA: the journal of the American Medical Association 13;292(14):1724–1737. Review. Erratum in: JAMA. 2005 13;293(14):1728

Heylen AM, Jacobs A, Lybeer M et al (2011) The OTSC®-clip in revisional endoscopy against weight gain after bariatric gastric bypass surgery Obes Surg 21:1629–1633

Mullady DK, Lautz DB, Thompson CC (2009) Treatment of weight regain after gastric bypass surgery when using a new endoscopic platform: initial experience and early outcomes (with video). Gastrointest Endosc 70:440–444

MIX
Papier aus verantwortungsvollen Quellen
Paper from responsible sources
FSC® C105338

If you have any concerns about our products,
you can contact us on
ProductSafety@springernature.com

In case Publisher is established outside the EU,
the EU authorized representative is:
Springer Nature Customer Service Center GmbH
Europaplatz 3, 69115 Heidelberg, Germany

Printed by Libri Plureos GmbH
in Hamburg, Germany